Spinal Cord Inj
Rehabilitation

T0259075

Editors

DIANA D. CARDENAS
KEVIN DALAL

PHYSICAL MEDICINE AND REHABILITATION CLINICS OF NORTH AMERICA

www.pmr.theclinics.com

Consulting Editor
GREGORY T. CARTER

August 2014 • Volume 25 • Number 3

ELSEVIER

1600 John F. Kennedy Boulevard ● Suite 1800 ● Philadelphia, Pennsylvania, 19103-2899

http://www.theclinics.com

PHYSICAL MEDICINE AND REHABILITATION CLINICS OF NORTH AMERICA Volume 25, Number 3
August 2014 ISSN 1047-9651, ISBN 978-0-323-32023-8

Editor: Jennifer Flynn-Briggs
Developmental Editor: Don Mumford

© **2014 Elsevier Inc. All rights reserved.**

This periodical and the individual contributions contained in it are protected under copyright by Elsevier, and the following terms and conditions apply to their use:

Photocopying
Single photocopies of single articles may be made for personal use as allowed by national copyright laws. Permission of the Publisher and payment of a fee is required for all other photocopying, including multiple or systematic copying, copying for advertising or promotional purposes, resale, and all forms of document delivery. Special rates are available for educational institutions that wish to make photocopies for non-profit educational classroom use. For information on how to seek permission visit www.elsevier.com/permissions or call: (+44) 1865 843830 (UK)/(+1) 215 239 3804 (USA).

Derivative Works
Subscribers may reproduce tables of contents or prepare lists of articles including abstracts for internal circulation within their institutions. Permission of the Publisher is required for resale or distribution outside the institution. Permission of the Publisher is required for all other derivative works, including compilations and translations (please consult www.elsevier.com/permissions).

Electronic Storage or Usage
Permission of the Publisher is required to store or use electronically any material contained in this periodical, including any article or part of an article (please consult www.elsevier.com/permissions). Except as outlined above, no part of this publication may be reproduced, stored in a retrieval system or transmitted in any form or by any means, electronic, mechanical, photocopying, recording or otherwise, without prior written permission of the Publisher.

Notice
No responsibility is assumed by the Publisher for any injury and/or damage to persons or property as a matter of products liability, negligence or otherwise, or from any use or operation of any methods, products, instructions or ideas contained in the material herein. Because of rapid advances in the medical sciences, in particular, independent verification of diagnoses and drug dosages should be made.

Although all advertising material is expected to conform to ethical (medical) standards, inclusion in this publication does not constitute a guarantee or endorsement of the quality or value of such product or of the claims made of it by its manufacturer.

Reprints. For copies of 100 or more of articles in this publication, please contact the Commercial Reprints Department, Elsevier Inc., 360 Park Avenue South, New York, NY 10010-1710. Tel.: 212-633-3874; Fax: 212-633-3820; E-mail: reprints@elsevier.com.

Physical Medicine and Rehabilitation Clinics of North America (ISSN 1047-9651) is published quarterly by Elsevier Inc., 360 Park Avenue South, New York, NY 10010-1710. Months of issue are February, May, August, and November. Business and Editorial Offices: 1600 John F. Kennedy Blvd., Suite 1800, Philadelphia, PA 19103-2899. Customer Service Office: 3251 Riverport Lane, Maryland Heights, MO 63043. Periodicals postage paid at New York, NY and additional mailing offices. Subscription price per year is $275.00 (US individuals), $486.00 (US institutions), $145.00 (US students), $335.00 (Canadian individuals), $640.00 (Canadian institutions), $210.00 (Canadian students), $415.00 (foreign individuals), $640.00 (foreign institutions), and $210.00 (foreign students). Foreign air speed delivery is included in all *Clinics* subscription prices. All prices are subject to change without notice. **POSTMASTER:** Send address changes to *Physical Medicine and Rehabilitation Clinics of North America*, Customer Service Office: Elsevier Health Sciences Division, Subscription Customer Service, 3251 Riverport Lane, Maryland Heights, MO 63043. **Customer Service: 1-800-654-2452 (US). From outside of the United States, call 314-447-8871. Fax: 314-447-8029. E-mail: JournalsCustomer Service-usa@elsevier.com (for print support); JournalsOnlineSupport-usa@elsevier.com (for online support).**

Physical Medicine and Rehabilitation Clinics of North America is indexed in *Excerpta Medica, MEDLINE/ PubMed (Index Medicus), Cinahl, and Cumulative Index to Nursing and Allied Health Literature.*

Contributors

CONSULTING EDITOR

GREGORY T. CARTER, MD, MS
Consulting Medical Editor, Medical Director, St Luke's Rehabilitation Institute, Spokane, Washington; University of Washington, School of Medicine, Seattle, Washington

EDITORS

DIANA D. CARDENAS, MD, MHA
Professor and Chair, Department of Physical Medicine and Rehabilitation, University of Miami-Miller School of Medicine; Chief of Service, Jackson Rehabilitation Hospital, Miami, Florida

KEVIN DALAL, MD
Assistant Professor, Department of Physical Medicine and Rehabilitation, University of Miami-Miller School of Medicine, Miami, Florida

AUTHORS

GEMAYARET ALVAREZ, MD
Assistant Professor, Department of Physical Medicine and Rehabilitation, University of Miami-Miller School of Medicine, Miami Florida

MUSA L. AUDU, PhD
Motion Study Laboratory, Advanced Platform Technology Center; Research Associate Professor, Department of Biomedical Engineering, Case Western Reserve University, Cleveland, Ohio

GREGORY E. BIGFORD, PhD
Department of Neurological Surgery; The Miami Project to Cure Paralysis, University of Miami-Miller School of Medicine, Miami, Florida

KATH BOGIE, DPhil
Senior Research Scientist, Medical Research Services (151W), Louis Stokes Cleveland VA Medical Center; Advanced Platform Technology Center; Assistant Professor, Departments of Orthopaedics and Biomedical Engineering, Case Western Reserve University, Cleveland, Ohio

DENNIS J. BOURBEAU, PhD
Research Investigator, Cleveland FES Center; Medical Research Services (151W), Louis Stokes Cleveland VA Medical Center, Cleveland, Ohio

STEVEN W. BROSE, DO
Assistant Professor, Department of Physical Medicine and Rehabilitation, Case Western Reserve University; Spinal Cord Injury Service (128W), Louis Stokes Cleveland VA Medical Center; Cleveland FES Center, Cleveland, Ohio; Ohio University Heritage College of Osteopathic Medicine, Athens, Ohio

K. MING CHAN, MD
Professor, Division of Physical Medicine and Rehabilitation, Centre for Neuroscience, University of Alberta, Edmonton, Alberta, Canada

SARAH R. CHANG, BS
Advanced Platform Technology Center; Department of Biomedical Engineering, Case Western Reserve University, Cleveland, Ohio

RACHEL E. COWAN, PhD
Department of Neurological Surgery; The Miami Project to Cure Paralysis, University of Miami-Miller School of Medicine, Miami, Florida

KEVIN DALAL, MD
Assistant Professor, Department of Physical Medicine and Rehabilitation, University of Miami-Miller School of Medicine, Miami, Florida

ANTHONY F. DIMARCO, MD
Professor of Physical Medicine and Rehabilitation; Professor of Physiology and Biophysics, Case Western Reserve University; Cleveland FES Center; Research Scientist, Rammelkamp Research Center, MetroHealth Medical Center, Cleveland, Ohio

SEAN DUKELOW, MD, PhD
Assistant Professor, Division of Physical Medicine and Rehabilitation, Department of Clinical Neurosciences; Hotchkiss Brain Institute, University of Calgary, Calgary, Alberta, Canada

ANASTASIA L. ELIAS, PhD
Assistant Professor, Chemical and Materials Engineering, University of Alberta, Edmonton, Alberta, Canada

ELIZABETH ROY FELIX, PhD
Research Assistant Professor, Department of Physical Medicine and Rehabilitation, University of Miami-Miller School of Medicine; Research Health Scientist, Research Service, Department of Veterans Affairs Medical Center, Miami VAHS, Miami, Florida

DEEP S. GARG, MD
Department of Physical Medicine and Rehabilitation, Jackson Memorial Hospital, University of Miami-Miller School of Medicine, Miami, Florida

LANCE L. GOETZ, MD
Staff Physician, Spinal Cord Injury Service, Department of Veterans Affairs, Hunter Holmes McGuire VA Medical Center; Associate Professor, Department of Physical Medicine and Rehabilitation, Virginia Commonwealth University, Richmond, Virginia

KENNETH J. GUSTAFSON, PhD
Associate Professor, Departments of Biomedical Engineering and Urology, Case Western Reserve University; Medical Research Services (151W), Louis Stokes Cleveland VA Medical Center; Cleveland FES Center, Cleveland, Ohio

CHESTER H. HO, MD
Associate Professor and Head, Division of Physical Medicine and Rehabilitation, Department of Clinical Neurosciences, Foothills Medical Centre; Hotchkiss Brain Institute, University of Calgary, Calgary, Alberta, Canada

ROBERT W. IRWIN, MD
Associate Chair for Education; Associate Professor, Department of Rehabilitation Medicine; Assistant Dean For Student Affairs, Medical Education, University of Miami-Miller School of Medicine, Miami, Florida

SEEMA R. KHURANA, DO
Assistant Professor, Department of Physical Medicine and Rehabilitation, University of Miami-Miller School of Medicine, Miami, Florida

KEVIN L. KILGORE, PhD
Medical Research Services (151W), Louis Stokes Cleveland VA Medical Center; Department of Biomedical Engineering, Case Western Reserve University; Cleveland FES Center; MetroHealth Medical Center, Cleveland, Ohio

STEVEN KIRSHBLUM, MD
Kessler Institute for Rehabilitation, West Orange, New Jersey; Rutgers New Jersey Medical School, Newark, New Jersey

ZELMA H.T. KISS, MD, PhD
Associate Professor, Director Neuromodulation Program; Division of Neurosurgery, Department of Clinical Neurosciences, Foothills Medical Centre; Hotchkiss Brain Institute, University of Calgary, Calgary, Alberta, Canada

ADAM P. KLAUSNER, MD
Staff Physician, Surgery Service, Department of Veterans Affairs, Hunter Holmes McGuire VA Medical Center; Associate Professor/Warren Koontz, Professor of Urologic Research, Division of Urology, Department of Surgery, Virginia Commonwealth University, Richmond, Virginia

RUDI KOBETIC, MS
Advanced Platform Technology Center, Medical Research Services, Louis Stokes Cleveland VA Medical Center, Cleveland, Ohio

JOCHEN KRESSLER, PhD
Department of Neurological Surgery; The Miami Project to Cure Paralysis, University of Miami-Miller School of Medicine, Miami, Florida

DAVID S. KUSHNER, MD
Associate Professor, Department of Physical Medicine and Rehabilitation, University of Miami-Miller School of Medicine, Miami, Florida

VIVIAN K. MUSHAHWAR, PhD
Professor, Division of Physical Medicine and Rehabilitation, Centre for Neuroscience, University of Alberta, Edmonton, Alberta, Canada

MARK S. NASH, PhD
Department of Neurological Surgery; The Miami Project to Cure Paralysis; Department of Rehabilitation Medicine, University of Miami-Miller School of Medicine, Miami, Florida

ANDREW L. SHERMAN, MD, MS
Department of Physical Medicine and Rehabilitation, University of Miami-Miller School of Medicine, Miami, Florida

GABRIEL SUNN, MD
Physical Medicine and Wound Rehabilitation, Spinal Cord Injury Unit, Miami VA Hospital; Voluntary Professor of Physical Medicine and Rehabilitation, University of Miami-Miller School of Medicine, Miami, Florida

RONALD J. TRIOLO, PhD
Senior Research Career Scientist, Louis Stokes Cleveland VA Medical Center; Executive Director, Advanced Platform Technology Center; Professor, Departments of Orthopaedics and Biomedical Engineering, Case Western Reserve University; MetroHealth Medical Center, Cleveland, Ohio

ALBERT H. VETTE, PhD
Assistant Professor, Department of Mechanical Engineering, University of Alberta; Glenrose Rehabilitation Hospital, Edmonton, Alberta, Canada

MICHAEL Y. WANG, MD, FACS
Department of Neurological Surgery, University of Miami-Miller School of Medicine, Miami, Florida

WILLIAM WARING III, MS, MD
Department of Physical Medicine and Rehabilitation, Medical College of Wisconsin, Milwaukee, Wisconsin

ERIN T. WOLFF, MD
Assistant Professor, Department of Rehabilitation Medicine, University of Miami-Miller School of Medicine, Miami, Florida

Contents

The International Standards for Neurological Classification of Spinal Cord Injury (ISNCSCI) is the most widely used classification in the field of spinal cord injury medicine. Since its first publication in 1982, multiple revisions refining the recommended examination, scaling, and classification have taken place to improve communication, consistency, and clarity. This article describes a brief historical perspective on the development and changes over the years leading to the current ISNCSCI, detailing the most recent updates of 2011 and the worksheet 2013 as well as issues facing the ISNCSCI for the future.

Applying therapeutic hypothermia (TH) for the purposes of neuroprotection, originally termed "hibernation," started nearly 100 years ago. Because TH cooling systems have improved to the point where it is practical and safe for general application, interest in providing such treatment in conditions such as spinal cord injury, traumatic brain injury, stroke, and cardiac arrest has increased. This article reviews the mechanisms by which TH mitigates secondary neurologic injury, the clinical scenarios where TH is being applied, and reviews selected published studies using TH for central nervous system neuroprotection.

Upper extremity pain in persons with spinal cord injury is a common cause of morbidity. Ultrasound of nerve, muscle, and tendon has the potential to become a valuable modality in assessing this population, and has the advantage of reduced health care costs, portability, and use in populations that cannot tolerate MRI. It has the potential to detect issues before the onset of significant morbidity, and preserve patient independence. Upper extremity ultrasound already has many studies showing its utility in diagnosis, and newer techniques have the potential to enhance its use in the diagnosis and management of musculoskeletal conditions.

Chronic neuropathic pain develops in approximately 40% of people after a spinal cord injury (SCI) and is notoriously difficult to treat. Because of the frequent presence of more than one pain type and the complex mechanisms and symptoms associated with pain in individuals with SCI, a thorough evaluation is important. This review includes an overview of the most recent guidelines for evaluating and classifying pain, suggestions for standardizing outcome measures for clinical use, and a review of the positive and negative evidence for pharmacologic and nonpharmacologic interventions to consider when treating individuals with SCI and chronic neuropathic pain.

Accelerated cardiometabolic disease is a serious health hazard after spinal cord injuries (SCI). Lifestyle intervention with diet and exercise remains the cornerstone of effective cardiometabolic syndrome treatment. Behavioral approaches enhance compliance and benefits derived from both diet and exercise interventions and are necessary to assure that persons with SCI profit from intervention. Multitherapy strategies will likely be needed to control challenging component risks, such as gain in body mass, which has far reaching implications for maintenance of daily function as well as health.

In this article, the problem of urinary tract infections (UTIs) after spinal cord injury and disorders is defined, the relationship of bladder management to UTIs is discussed, and mechanical and medical strategies for UTI prevention in spinal cord injury and disorders are described.

After cervical spinal cord injuries, many patients are unable to sustain independent ventilation because of a disruption of diaphragm innervation and respiratory functioning. If phrenic nerve function is preserved, the patient may be able to tolerate exogenous pacing of the diaphragm via electrical stimulation. Previously this was accomplished by stimulation directly to the phrenic nerves, but may be accomplished less invasively by percutaneously stimulating the diaphragm itself. The benefits, when compared with mechanical ventilation, include a lower rate of pulmonary complications, improved venous return, more normal breathing and speech, facilitation of eating, cost-effectiveness, and increased patient mobility.

Chester H. Ho, Ronald J. Triolo, Anastasia L. Elias, Kevin L. Kilgore,
Anthony F. DiMarco, Kath Bogie, Albert H. Vette, Musa L. Audu,
Rudi Kobetic, Sarah R. Chang, K. Ming Chan, Sean Dukelow,
Dennis J. Bourbeau, Steven W. Brose, Kenneth J. Gustafson,
Zelma H.T. Kiss, and Vivian K. Mushahwar

Spinal cord injuries (SCI) can disrupt communications between the brain and the body, resulting in loss of control over otherwise intact neuromuscular systems. Functional electrical stimulation (FES) of the central and peripheral nervous system can use these intact neuromuscular systems to provide therapeutic exercise options to allow functional restoration and to manage medical complications following SCI. The use of FES for the restoration of muscular and organ functions may significantly decrease the morbidity and mortality following SCI. Many FES devices are commercially available and should be considered as part of the lifelong rehabilitation care plan for all eligible persons with SCI.

Seema R. Khurana and Deep S. Garg

Muscle spasms and spasticity constitute a significant problem in patients with spinal cord injury, interfering with rehabilitation and leading to impairments in quality of life in addition to medical complications. Administration of intrathecal baclofen (ITB) is indicated when spasticity continues to produce a clinical disability despite trials of oral treatments and other alternatives in patients who have functional goals and/or pain without contractures. Severe spasticity of spinal origin has been shown to respond dramatically to long-term ITB when used in appropriate patients with spasticity.

Gabriel Sunn

Pressure ulcers continue to impact the lives of spinal cord injury patients severely. Pressure ulcers must be accurately staged according to National Pressure Ulcer Advisory recommendations before treatment design. The first priority in treatment of pressure ulcers is offloading. Intact skin ulcers may be treated with noncontact nonthermal low-frequency ultrasound. Superficial pressure ulcers may be treated with a combination of collagenase and foam dressings. Deeper pressure ulcers warrant negative-pressure wound therapy dressings along with biologic adjuncts to fill in wound depth. Discovery and treatment of osteomyelitis is a high priority when initially evaluating pressure ulcers. Surgical intervention must always be considered.

David S. Kushner and Gemayaret Alvarez

Spinal cord injury (SCI) patients should be assessed for a co-occurring traumatic brain injury (TBI) on admission to a rehabilitation program. Incidence of a dual diagnosis may approach 60% with certain risk factors. Diagnosis of mild–moderate severity TBIs may be missed during acute care hospitalizations of SCI. Neuropsychological symptoms of a missed TBI diagnosis may be perceived during rehabilitation as noncompliance, inability to learn, maladaptive reactions to SCI, and poor motivation. There are life-threatening and quality-of-life–threatening complications of TBI that also may be missed if a dual diagnosis is not made.

PHYSICAL MEDICINE & REHABILITATION CLINICS OF NORTH AMERICA

VISIT THE CLINICS ONLINE!
Access your subscription at:
www.theclinics.com

PHYSICAL MEDICINE & REHABILITATION CLINICS OF NORTH AMERICA

FORTHCOMING ISSUES

November 2014
Sports Medicine
Brian J. Krabak, Editor

February 2015
Pediatric Rehabilitation
Andrew Skalsky, Editor

RECENT ISSUES

May 2014
Challenging Pain Syndromes
Adam L. Schreiber, Editor

February 2014
Amputee Rehabilitation
Robert H. Meier III, Editor

November 2013
Multiple Sclerosis Rehabilitation
Shana L. Johnson and
George H. Kraft, Editor

August 2013
Life Care Planning
Michel Lacerte and
Cloie B. Johnson, Editor

RELATED INTEREST ISSUES

Neuroimaging Clinics, May 2014 (Vol. 24, Issue 2)
The Postoperative Spine: What the Spine Surgeon Needs to Know
Orlando M. Airitano, Alexandre S. de Moura, and Ruby J. Lien, Editor

Neurologic Clinics, February 2013 (Vol. 31, Issue 1)
Spine and Spinal Cord Trauma: Diagnosis and Management
Shlomo Zhang, Robin Wachawa, Julio D. Heydel, Jonas Tony, Kendric Johnson, and Bruce L. Gieftheode, Editor

Clinics in Sports Medicine, July 2012 (Vol. 31, Issue 3)
Spinal Cord Abnormalities in Sports
Mark R. Proctor and R. Michael Scott, Editor

VISIT THE CLINICS ONLINE!
Access your subscription at:
www.theclinics.com

Foreword

Spinal Cord Injury Rehabilitation

 CrossMark

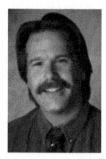

Gregory T. Carter, MD, MS
Consulting Editor

As someone who has spent the vast majority of his career in the Pacific Northwest, when we decided to do an updated issue on spinal cord injury (SCI) rehabilitation, I immediately thought of my friend and colleague, Dr Diana Cardenas. When Dr Cardenas was here at the University of Washington, she developed and directed a nationally recognized SCI Center of Excellence. This was the "go to" place for all of us to refer our SCI patients for their annual complete evaluation and checkup. For many years now, Dr Cardenas has served as Professor and Chair, Department of Rehabilitation Medicine and Chief of Service and Medical Director, Department of Rehabilitation Medicine at the University of Miami Miller School of Medicine. She is also part of the Miami Project to Cure Paralysis (the Buoniconti Fund).

As I suspected she would, Dr Cardenas recruited a list of "who's who" in spinal cord medicine to author the articles within this issue.

This issue starts with an excellent article entitled, "Updates for the International Standards for Neurological Classification of Spinal Cord Injury (ISNCSCI)," by Drs Kirshblum and Waring. This is a great overview and provides an excellent treatise on how to use these standards to improve care.

Drs Goetz and Klausner authored, "Strategies for Prevention of Urinary Tract Infections in Neurogenic Bladder Dysfunction," which provides up-to-date strategies on how to approach and treat this significant problem seen in the vast majority of patients of SCI and neurogenic bladder.

Moving into a more experimental topic, Drs Sherman and Wang present, "Hypothermia as a Clinical Neuroprotectant." As they point out, there is now a very robust body of experimental evidence that hypothermia is beneficial in the treatment of acute SCI. The potential benefits of hypothermia in preventing or limiting SCI following trauma are discussed in detail along with an overview of the potential use of hypothermia after SCI.

Phys Med Rehabil Clin N Am 25 (2014) xiii–xiv
http://dx.doi.org/10.1016/j.pmr.2014.07.001
1047-9651/14/$ – see front matter © 2014 Elsevier Inc. All rights reserved.

Dr Dalal offers an excellent overview of "Diaphragmatic Pacing in Spinal Cord Injury." In this article, there is first-rate coverage of the problem of chronic hypoventilation that can be seen in higher injury level quadriplegics. Diaphragm pacing through electrical stimulation of the phrenic nerve can be a very effective treatment for central hypoventilation syndrome in patients with SCI, and the article by Dr Dalal discusses the use of phrenic nerve stimulation for diaphragm pacing to address this.

Drs Kushner and Alvarez have co-authored, "Dual Diagnosis: Traumatic Brain Injury with Spinal Cord Injury." This exceptional article overviews and interprets the research into the problems encountered by people with SCI and coexistent or traumatic brain injury, which may often be overlooked. Patients with concomitant SCI and traumatic brain injury often present unique challenges and this article fully explores that.

Drs Kressler, Cowen, Bigford, and Nash present an excellent treatise on "Reducing Cardiometabolic Disease in Spinal Cord Injury," which is a major secondary cause of comorbidity given the impaired ability to exercise for patients with SCI.

"Chronic Neuropathic Pain in SCI: Evaluation and Treatment" is authored by Dr Felix, a noted expert in this area. Neuropathic pain is a known consequence of SCI and may persist for years after the inciting injury. Dr Felix gives recommendations for diagnostic and treatment strategies for this problem, including a discussion of the use of anticonvulsant agents, tricyclic antidepressants, and other strategies.

An outstanding discussion on "Spasticity and the Use of Intrathecal Baclofen in Patients with Spinal Cord Injury" is provided by Drs Khurana and Garg, followed by a very thorough article authored by Drs Irwin and Wolff, entitled, "Assessment of Neuromuscular Conditions Using Ultrasound."

This issue concludes with an article entitled, "Functional Electrical Stimulation and Spinal Cord Injury," by Drs Ho, Triolo, Elias, Kilgore, DiMarco, Bogie, Vette, Audu, Kobetic, Chang, Chan, Dukelow, Bourbeau, Brose, Gustafson, Kiss, and Mushawar, and an article entitled, "Spinal Cord Injury Pressure Ulcer Treatment: An Evidence-based Approach," by Dr Sunn. These are both outstanding articles.

I want to thank all of these distinguished authors, and in particular, our editors, Drs Cardenas and Dalal, for giving us such a wonderful, up-to-date, and remarkably thorough issue on SCI rehabilitation. These authors have given us a directly useful and highly valuable addition to the *Physical Medicine and Rehabilitation Clinics of North America* series.

Gregory T. Carter, MD, MS
St Luke's Rehabilitation Institute
711 South Cowley Street
Spokane, WA 99202, USA

E-mail address:
gtcarter@uw.edu

Preface

Spinal Cord Injury Rehabilitation

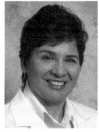 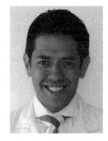

Diana D. Cardenas, MD, MHA   Kevin Dalal, MD

Editors

I would like to thank Gregory Carter, MD, for inviting me to be a guest editor for a *Physical Medicine and Rehabilitation Clinics of North America* issue on Spinal Cord Injury (SCI) Medicine. Kevin Dalal, MD, medical director of the SCI unit at Jackson Rehabilitation Hospital, Miami, Florida, has the clinical "hands-on" experience and the up-to-date knowledge in SCI to ably fill the role of coeditor. Together, we have presented what we hope will be one of the best issues in the series. Our goal is to include a range of topics in SCI from acute neuroprotection to chronic complications, focusing on some of the technological advances that have informed specific areas. The topics selected for in-depth discussion are those whose management protocols may not be typically available in more general physical medicine and rehabilitation resources or that involve new strategies.

Fundamental to our ability to provide care to our patients, educate our medical students and trainees, and conduct SCI clinical research is having well-defined standards for neurological classification based on the clinical examination. The first article, therefore, reviews the International Standards for Neurological Classification of SCI, known since 2000 as the "ISNCSCI." The ISNCSCI has evolved over time in the hopes of giving a precise and easily duplicated assessment of such injuries. Also discussed is the ASIA Impairment Scale and the recent educational modules that address standards for autonomic function and spasticity.

Technological advances are the topics for articles on the use of hypothermia as a clinical neuroprotectant to blunt the inflammatory cascade that contributes to SCI, the use of ultrasound to diagnose acute and chronic neuromuscular issues in SCI, and the use of functional electrical stimulation for respiration, upper and lower extremity function, and bladder function. Phrenic nerve electrical stimulation has been used for decades. More recently, less invasive surgical techniques have developed that have increased the potential number of patients with high-level tetraplegia, complete or

Phys Med Rehabil Clin N Am 25 (2014) xv–xvi
http://dx.doi.org/10.1016/j.pmr.2014.06.001
1047-9651/14/$ – see front matter © 2014 Published by Elsevier Inc.

pmr.theclinics.com

incomplete, who may be candidates for a diaphragm pacemaker, a device that can obviate long-term ventilator management and its associated costs and care burden.

As the length of stay for inpatient rehabilitation shortens and care shifts to outpatient practice, two nearly universal concerns that deserve discussion include neuropathic pain and spasticity management. The pathways and management strategies for these conditions are discussed in respective articles as well. Other common causes of morbidity in spinal cord–injured patients include neurogenic bladder (and associated UTIs) and pressure ulcer development. Given their prevalence and impact on the spinal cord population, their discussion is an integral part of any collection of SCI management topics. Issues with a more longitudinal impact as the spinal cord–injured population ages and has ever-improving longevity include obesity and cardiovascular disease. We know that cardiovascular disease is a leading cause of mortality and we have included a discussion of management of both obesity and cardiovascular disease in this issue.

Finally, the discussion of the dual diagnosis of SCI and traumatic brain injury is an important consideration as many trauma patients with SCI may be underdiagnosed with both conditions, and such patients may require a more careful focus of care.

Each of the authors selected to present a topic has vast knowledge and experience in their respective field of discussion, and their contributions will further assist in bringing new recommendations and reinforcing treatment guidelines to manage many challenging aspects of SCI. We hope that you will find this issue of practical value and perhaps even new research ideas will be generated.

Diana D. Cardenas, MD, MHA
Department of Physical Medicine and Rehabilitation
University of Miami Miller School of Medicine
Miami, FL 33136, USA

Jackson Rehabilitation Hospital
Miami, FL 33136, USA

Kevin Dalal, MD
Department of Physical Medicine and Rehabilitation
University of Miami Miller School of Medicine
Miami, FL 33101, USA

E-mail addresses:
DCardenas@med.miami.edu (D.D. Cardenas)
kdalal@med.miami.edu (K. Dalal)

Updates for the International Standards for Neurological Classification of Spinal Cord Injury

CrossMark

Steven Kirshblum, MD[a,b,*], William Waring III, MS, MD[c]

KEYWORDS

- Spinal cord injury • International Standards • Classification • Neurologic level

KEY POINTS

- The latest changes to the International Standards for Neurological Classification of Spinal Cord Injury (ISNCSCI) were made in 2011 and 2013.
- The purpose of the ISNCSCI remains to allow for accurate communication between clinicians and researchers working in the field of spinal cord injury (SCI).
- The ISNCSCI continues to evolve based on feedback from professionals in SCI.

HISTORICAL BACKGROUND AND REVISIONS

Accurate communication between clinicians and researchers working with SCI patients requires that standards be used in the classification of neurologic impairment.[1] Such a standardized method is important to help document the course of recovery and the effect of interventions in the treatment of SCI, including regeneration.[2] To this end, the American Spinal Injury Association (ASIA) first developed and published the *Standards For Neurological Classification Of Spinal Injury Patients* in 1982,[1] which has since become the most widely used classification in the field.

Prior to this, in an attempt for consistency of definitions in 1969, a questionnaire was completed by leading physicians in the field of SCI to establish international agreement on neurologic terminology for SCI and to compare their opinions on the best time to accurately predict outcome after SCI. Their recommendations were

This article was supported in part by the National Institute on Disability and Rehabilitation Research (grant no. H133N060022).
[a] Kessler Institute for Rehabilitation, Rutgers New Jersey Medical School, West Orange, NJ 07052, USA; [b] Rutgers New Jersey Medical School, Newark, NJ, USA; [c] Department of Physical Medicine and Rehabilitation, Medical College of Wisconsin, 9200 Wisconsin Avenue, Milwaukee, WI 53226, USA
* Corresponding author.
E-mail address: skirshblum@kessler-rehab.com

1047-9651/14/$ – see front matter © 2014 Elsevier Inc. All rights reserved.

published, but there was no agreement on the overall classification of SCI.[3] Several classifications for SCI were subsequently proposed based on bony patterns of injury, mechanism of injury, neurologic function, and functional outcome.[4–10] In 1969, Frankel and colleagues[11] described a 5-grade system of classifying traumatic SCI, with a division into complete (A) and 4 incomplete (B–E) injury grades. The purpose of this article was to describe results of postural reduction in the treatment of SCI, and they described their classification as "crude." ASIA's first booklet of the *Standards For Neurological Classification Of Spinal Injury Patients*,[1] published in 1982, incorporated the Frankel grades A–E along with an introduction of motor testing of key muscle groups and sensory testing in 29 dermatomes. These standards defined or described the following:

- Clarification of injury based on neurologic complete and incomplete injuries based on sparing below the level of injury
- Neurologic zone of injury (NLI)
- Quadriplegia, quadraperesis, paraplegia, and paraparesis
- Zone of injury up to 3 neurologic segments at the point of damage to the spinal cord where there is frequently some preservation of motor and/or sensory function
- Anatomic incomplete clinical syndromes (eg, central cord syndrome [CCS])

The standards from 1982 were refined by ASIA over the next 10 years, involving input from SCI clinicians and researchers.[12–15] Changes included the use of specific key areas with anatomic landmarks to define the sensory level, combining the S4 and S5 dermatomes into a single S4-5 dermatome (perianal area), reducing the total number of dermatomes to 28, and redefining the zone of injury as the zone of partial preservation (ZPP) of sensory and/or motor function. Other changes included having only the elbow flexors examined to test the C5 myotome, clarification of muscle grading in the determination of motor levels, and clarification of the Frankel classification in terms of the degree of incompleteness (Frankel grade C vs D) as recommended by Tator and colleagues.[13] Use of the terms, *quadraparesis* and *paraparesis*, was discouraged because they imprecisely described incomplete lesions.

In 1992, the fourth revision of the ISNCSCI was published.[16] The key change of this major revision was the replacement of the Frankel classification with the ASIA Impairment Scale (AIS), with a major change in adopting the sacral sparing definition to determine the completeness of the injury. The sacral sparing definition of the completeness of the injury was considered a more stable definition, because fewer patients convert from incomplete to complete status over time postinjury.[17] The AIS, similar to the Frankel scale, described 5 different severities of SCI. Other features of the 1992 revision included

- Incorporating the Functional Independence Measure (FIM)
- Printing of the key sensory points
- Testing pinprick and light touch separately on a 3-point scale
- Sensory index scoring
- Motor level changed such that a grade 4 on testing was no longer considered normal, unless it was examiner judgment that certain inhibiting factors, such as pain, positioning of the patient, hypertonicity, or disuse inhibited full effort
- Modification of the definition of the ZPP
- Optional tests (position sense, vibration, and additional muscles to better localize the level of the lesion) were added
- *Tetraplegia* introduced, as preferred to the term, *quadriplegia*.

These standards were endorsed by the International Medical Society of Paraplegia and, thereafter, became known as the "International Standards for Neurological and Functional Classification of Spinal Cord Injury."[16]

In 1994, ASIA published a written manual for the ISNCSCI and videos of the examination.[18] To the 1996 version of the ISNCSCI booklet included clarification of how to score muscles whose strength may be affected by inhibiting factors and further clarification of how to differentiate between AIS C and D plus instructions on how to determine the motor level when the sensory level falls into a region where the key muscles cannot be clinically tested; for C1-C4, T2-L1, and S3-5, the motor level is designated as the same as the most rostral normal sensory level.[19]

The revisions to the ISNCSCI in 2000[20] further clarified motor incomplete injuries and how to document the ZPP and eliminated the FIM from the standards. This revision developed the now current title, *The International Standards for the Neurological Classification of Spinal Cord Injury*. In 2003, ASIA published a revised version of the written manual for the ISNCSCI.[21] Additional minor revisions and reprintings of the booklet were published in 2002, 2006, and 2008. In 2006, ASIA started developing an Internet-based learning course for the ISNCSCI, called the International Standards Training eLearning Program (InSTeP) that is available and continues to be updated along with the ISNCSCI. InSTeP offers modules on anatomy as well as how to perform an examination and classify an injury based on the AIS.[22] In 2009 an update was published to explain some of the updates and processes of the International Standards Committee.[23]

2011 REVISIONS OF THE ISNCSCI

In 2011, the seventh revision of the ISNCSCI was published,[24] along with an accompanying explanatory article,[25] and included some clarifications as well as changes that were substantial enough such that the 2003 reference manual was no longer to be used or distributed.

The clarifications of the 2011 revisions included

1. Greater detail describing the motor and sensory examination, including positions for motor testing, reinforcing specific manual muscle techniques, using static positioning with a patient resisting the examiner's force, to grade a muscle function as 4 or 5.[24] It was thought that standardization in performing muscle testing would allow for consistency in grading among examiners. Details on execution of the examination are available as part of the InSTeP program[22] and **Box 1** lists the specific positions for testing key muscles for grades 4 and 5.[23]
2. When defining the motor level in a patient with no correlating key motor function to test (above C5, between T2 and L1, and between S2 and S5), the motor level is presumed the same as the sensory level, if testable motor function above (rostral) that level is intact (normal) as well. Based on sample testing, it was thought that this concept required clarification, and examples were used to illustrate this point (**Box 2**).
3. When documenting the ZPP on the worksheet in a case that there is no sparing of motor or sensory function below the motor and sensory levels, the relevant (right and left) motor and sensory levels are placed in the designated area on the worksheet. Previously, it was not clear what should be documented in the worksheet box when the motor and/or sensory level was the same as the NLI without any distal sparing. It was also clarified that motor function does not follow sensory function in recording ZPP. Rather, the caudal extent of the motor ZPP is based only on the presence of voluntary muscle function below the motor level. Although the

---

Box 1
Positions for testing key muscles for grade 4 or 5

C5: Elbow flexed at 90°, arm at patient's side, and forearm supinated

C6: Wrist in full extension

C7: Shoulder in neutral rotation, adducted, and in 90° of flexion, with elbow in 45° of flexion

C8: Full flexed position of the distal phalanx with the proximal finger joints stabilized in extended position

T1: Full abducted position of fifth digit (of the hand)

L2: Hip flexed to 90°

L3: Knee flexed to 15°

L4: Full dorsiflexed position of ankle

L5: First toe fully extended

S1: Hip in neutral rotation, the knee is fully extended and the ankle in full plantarflexion.

From Kirshblum SC, Waring W, Biering-Sorensen F, et al. Reference for the 2011 revision of the International Standards for Neurological Classification of Spinal Cord Injury. J Spinal Cord Med 2011;34(6):548; with permission.

---

motor level defers to the sensory level in the regions where there is no key motor function to test (C1-C4, T2-L1, and so forth), motor ZPP does not defer to the sensory ZPP. Specifically, if the NLI is T6 in a case with a neurologically complete injury (AIS A), with impaired sparing of light touch sensation at T7 bilaterally and all other sensations absent, T7 should be documented for sensation bilaterally and T6 for the motor ZPP bilaterally.

4. To distinguish between a sensory incomplete versus a motor incomplete (AIS B from C) injury, the motor level on each side is used, whereas the single neurologic level is used to distinguish motor incomplete injuries (AIS C from D). This concept was previously documented but was still found to cause some confusion.

5. Non key muscle functions may be used to determine sensory versus motor incomplete status (AIS B vs C) as previously alluded to in 2003.[21] This was thought important because the presence of motor function in a non key muscle, in a sensory incomplete scenario below the motor level could represent a motor incomplete injury and as such offer a significant difference in potential recovery, for inclusion/exclusion criteria for research studies, or as an outcome measure in a trial designed to restore strength in persons with motor complete injuries. Specific levels for non key muscles were further delineated in 2013 to assure consistency of how these findings were used (discussed later).

The 2011 new changes to the ISNCSCI include

1. Replacing the term, *deep anal sensation*, with the term, *deep anal pressure (DAP)*. Consensus determined that the term, *pressure*, reinforced the technique of applying gentle pressure to the anorectal wall with an examiner's distal thumb and index finger[26] as opposed to other more vigorous techniques that may potentially relay information by other neurologic pathways (eg, autonomic) or eliciting visceral or somatic reflex activity.

2. If sensation is abnormal at C2, the level that should be designated is C1. This was documented because previous versions of the ISNCSCI did not include directions on the classification if C2 sensation was abnormal.

Box 2
Examples of motor level differing to the sensory level

Example 1: If the sensory level is C4, and there is no C5 motor strength (or the strength is graded <3), the motor level is C4.

Example 2: If the sensory level is C4, with the C5 key muscle function strength graded as ≥3, the motor level is C5. This is because the strength at C5 is ≥3 with the muscle function above considered normal. Presumably, if there were a C4 key muscle function, it is graded as normal because the sensation at C4 is intact.

Example 3: If the sensory level is C3, with the C5 key muscle function strength graded as ≥3, the motor level is C3. This is because the motor level presumably at C4 is not considered normal (because the C4 dermatome is not normal), and the rule of all levels rostral needing to be intact is not met.

Example 4: If all upper limb key muscle functions are intact, with intact sensation through T6, the sensory level as well as the motor level is recorded as T6.

Example 5: In a case similar to Example 4, but the T1 muscle function grade 3 instead of 5, whereas T6 is still the sensory level, the motor level is T1, because all the muscles above the T6 level cannot be considered normal. It is important to recognize that the motor level follows the sensory level only if the rule, "all the key muscle functions above are graded as normal," applies.

Example 6: If the sensory level is T12, the hip flexor motor function (L2 key muscle) is graded as 3 bilaterally and muscle strength of upper extremity key muscle groups are graded 5/5, the motor level is T12. Although L2 motor function is graded as a 3, the motor function above that level (L1) is not normal because the sensory level, and thereby the motor level, is T12.

Example 7: If the sensory level is L2 and the hip flexor muscle function is graded as a 2 with all upper extremity key motor function graded as 5, the sensory level is L2, and the motor level is L1. Although the rule of the motor level deferring to sensory level is used when there is no functional motor level to test (ie, above the L2 level), once there is a key motor functional level to test (in this case at L2), the motor level no longer defers to the sensory level.

From Kirshblum SC, Waring W, Biering-Sorensen F, et al. Reference for the 2011 revision of the International Standards for Neurological Classification of Spinal Cord Injury. J Spinal Cord Med 2011;34(6):548–9; with permission.

---

3. For clinical purposes in determining an AIS classification, in patients who have light touch or pinprick sensation at S4-5, examination for DAP is not required. Although testing for DAP was still recommended to complete the worksheet, its performance in this scenario would not change the classification because the patient already met the criteria for a sensory incomplete injury. In this situation, a digital rectal examination is still required for determining the presence of voluntary anal sphincter contraction.

4. The definition of ZPP in patients with a neurologically complete injury (AIS A) was revised to be consistent with InSTeP. The method used to determine the levels of the ZPP was changed to include the "dermatomes and myotomes caudal to the sensory and motor levels on each side of the body that remain partially innervated" in a neurologically complete patient. In the previous edition of the ISNCSCI prior to 2011, the ZPP was determined from the NLI. This distinction is important when discussing the levels of sparing for the ZPP.[23]

5. Several figures and the worksheet were updated. Updates on the worksheet included changing deep anal sensation to DAP, the addition of a box to enter the single neurologic level, and a definition printed for the ZPP.

2013 WORKSHEET

Based on recommendation from SCI professionals, an updated worksheet was presented at the ASIA conference in April 2013. The following items were added or adjusted to the worksheet (**Fig. 1**).

On page 1 of the worksheet:

1. At the top on the left, the abbreviation, ISNCSCI, was added.
2. Signature line was placed at the top on the right side of the page.
3. Dermatomal map was placed in the middle of the page. Previously it was on the right side of the page.
4. There is a right/left separation of motor and sensory scores on either side of the dermatomal map.
5. There is now alignment of motor and sensory levels (previously the motor and sensory levels were not aligned and caused some confusion).
6. There is now an increase of the size of the boxes for scoring of 15% to allow additional room for documentation. A larger increase would not allow the scores to fit on 1 page.
7. There is now shading of the column for pinprick scores (10% shading) to differentiate from light touch but still allowing for photocopying without the copy being distorted.
8. There is now alignment of sacral sparing components (voluntary anal contraction, DAP, and light touch and pinprick sensation at S4-5 levels) and bolded to allow for easy identification of sacral sparing.
9. There are now separate boxes for motor subscores (UEMS vs LEMS) because this is often used in clinical and research purposes.
10. A box was added to document the NLI.
11. Each of the boxes for the levels (eg, motor level and sensory level) was numbered, corresponding with directions on page 2 as to the steps to determine the AIS classification.

On page 2 of the worksheet:

1. Under the section, "Steps to Classification," for item #3—"Determine the single neurologic level," wording was adjusted to be consistent with the definitions. Specifically, instead of what was previously stated on the previous worksheet, "This is the lowest segment where motor and sensory function is normal on both sides, and is the most cephalad of the sensory and motor levels determined...", the wording was changed to, "This refers to the most caudal segment of the cord with intact sensation and antigravity (3 or more) muscle function strength, provided that there is normal (intact) sensation and motor function rostrally respectively."
2. The International Spinal Cord Society logo was placed on both sides of the form.
3. There is an addition of levels for non key muscles.

NON KEY MUSCLES

In 2003, it was documented that "non-key muscles can be used to determine between AIS B versus C."[21] Specifically, this allowed the use of non key muscles more than 3 levels below the motor level in a case scenario of a sensory incomplete injury to classify a patient with a motor incomplete injury. There was no documentation or consistency, however, regarding what levels should be used for the non key muscles. The specific levels are important, because 2 examiners can obtain

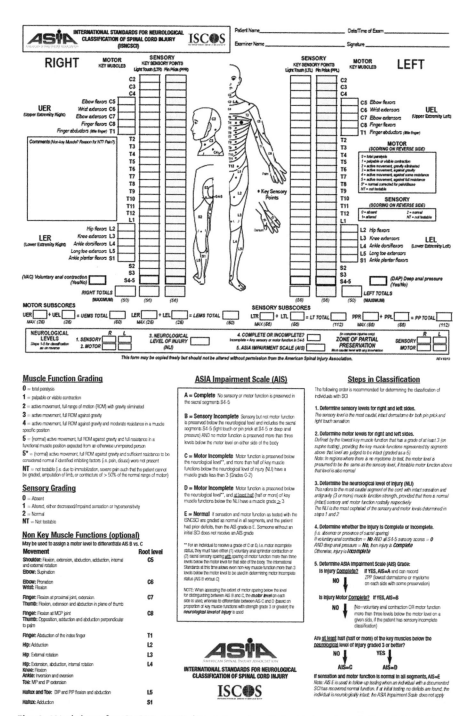

Fig. 1. Worksheet for ISNCSCI, 2013. (*From* American Spinal Injury Association: International Standards for Neurological Classification of Spinal Cord Injury, revised 2013; Atlanta, GA. Reprinted 2013; used with permission.)

the same motor scores for a specific muscle function, but if using different non key muscle functional levels, they may classify the patient differently. An example is a case scenario of a motor level of C5 with sensory sacral sparing and movement of the thumb (as a non key muscle function). If thumb movement is considered a C8 level function, then the AIS classification is AIS B, whereas if the movement of the thumb is considered a T1 function, then the classification is an AIS C (because T1 is more than 3 levels below the motor level, meeting criteria for a motor incomplete injury). Therefore, to allow for consistency of classification, levels were assigned for a majority of muscle functional activities in the upper and lower extremities (**Table 1**).

Motor levels were determined by reviewing multiple key reference sources for myotomal distributions of each of the non key muscles in the upper and lower extremities. From these, the most rostral (proximal) innervation of muscles that usually performs that activity was chosen. The list was reviewed by a neuroanatomist and then reviewed and approved by the committee. Functional movements were included in the table as opposed to specific muscles, to remove the potential difficult task of determining which of the possible muscles that can provide that function is active in each individual case.

Non key muscles are not recommended to be examined as a routine part of the ISNCSCI examination. Rather, they may be tested in cases in a patient with a presentation of a sensory incomplete injury (AIS B). There is no standardized technique as yet describing how to examine non key muscles and how to detect muscle substitutions resulting in false positives.

Table 1
Non key muscle groups

Movement	Root Level
Shoulder: flexion, extension, abduction, adduction, internal and external rotation Elbow: supination	C5
Elbow: pronation Wrist: flexion	C6
Finger: flexion at proximal joint, extension Thumb: flexion, extension, and abduction in plane of thumb	C7
Finger: flexion at MCP joint Thumb: opposition, adduction, and abduction perpendicular to palm	C8
Finger: abduction of little finger	T1
Hip: adduction	L2
Hip: ext rotation	L3
Hip: extension, abduction, int rotation Knee: flexion Ankle: inversion and eversion Toe: MP and IP extension	L4
Hallux and toe: DIP and PIP flexion and abduction	L5
Hallux: adduction	S1

Abbreviations: DIP, distal inter-phalangeal; Ext, external; Int, internal; MCP, metacarpo-phalangeal; PIP, proximal inter-phalangeal.

From ASIA e-Learning center. Available at: www.asia-spinalinjury.org/elearning/elearning.php. Accessed May 16, 2014; with permission.

FUTURE ISSUES FOR THE ISNCSCI

The ISNCSCI have changed over the years and ASIA International Standards Committee continues to strive to meet the needs for the field of SCI professionals. Although the preference is to have as few changes as possible, several issues are being reviewed to develop potential improvements for the future that may improve the classification to meet the needs of clinicians and researchers in SCI. Following are some of the important considerations being discussed.

Use of Computerized Algorithms

The classification of impairment is an independent skill from the performance of an examination and takes a great deal of understanding of the rules and nuances. As such, error rate of manual classification by trained professionals has been reported at approximately 10% in difficult cases.[27] Algorithms have been described[28–30] and, to date, 2 have become widely available online: the European Multicenter Study about Spinal Cord Injury[31] and the Rick Hansen Institute algorithms.[32] Both have been validated on large number of cases, are easily integrated into other software projects, use logic to deal with nontestable regions, and have been updated based on the 2011 ISNCSCI.

The benefits of algorithms may include consistency for classification of cases, ease of data review, 1-step clinical and data bank entry, facilitating documenting of non-SCI motor and sensory deficits, and eliminating the need for paper data collection forms with electronic medical records. Exceptions to the rules are often seen by clinicians that can have an impact on a variety of areas such as making an AIS classification, determining a medico-legal diagnosis, and potentially inclusion or exclusion into clinical trials. An example includes a patient with weakness and sensory deficits from a non–SCI-related injury (eg, brachial plexus injury) with an otherwise T6 level injury. A computerized algorithm could use the motor score of less than normal in the upper extremity to classify the patient as having a cervical level injury, while a SCI expert would recognize that the deficits were secondary to non–SCI-related injury (based on the comments made in the appropriate section on the worksheet) and, as such, appropriately classify the patient with the thoracic level.[23] A recent article discusses some challenging cases that clarify some of the confusion of the ISNCSCI but also included a case of chronic paraplegia with a new cervical SCI that a panel of expert could not reach.[33] Unless programmed for every exception, a computer algorithm may not be able to correctly classify all SCI's. On the other hand, creating a rule for every exception for a computer program flies against the reality that the current Standards are already very challenging to teach even to experts as evidenced by all of the extensive teaching/training activities. Ongoing discussion in ASIA Standards' Committee might address how to account for non-SCI related motor and sensory above the NLI but there are no plans or inclination to make new rules for every unusual SCI case. One recommendations to balance the utility of computer algorithm and clinical judgment with the ISNCSCI is to follow the model used with computerized ECG analysis that uses computerized algorithms that are only accepted after review by a expert provider.

Defining Incomplete Syndromes

Historically, the definitions of the commonly used incomplete syndromes, including CCS, Brown-Séquard syndrome, anterior cord syndrome, and others, have been included in the ISNCSCI booklets, but their use has not been recommended for classification partially due to the realization that not all cases fit into injury syndromes, and there is often a lack of clear guidelines for their use. For example, there is no consensus for differentiating between cases of incomplete tetraplegia from CCS in terms of, for example, a difference of the upper and lower extremities motor scores.[34,35] A clear definition is important, especially if the expectation is for a computerized program to be able to determine this classification. A similar issue is present for Brown-Séquard–like syndromes, because many patients have variations of the true description.[36]

Issues Relating to Deferring to the Sensory Level

The current ISNCSCI state that for those myotomes that are not clinically testable by manual muscle examination (eg, above C4, between T2 and T12, and below S1), the motor level is presumed the same as the sensory level if testable motor function above (rostral) that level is normal as well.[22] For example, in a case scenario where the C5 myotome has a grade greater than or equal to 3 and the sensory level is at C4, the motor level is C5. This is explained by the normal scoring for sensory at C4 that suggests that the motor level at C4, if testable, is also intact. Therefore, the rule of the motor level being a level that grades at least a 3, with the levels above it being normal, is met.

In a more difficult case scenario, however, where muscle testing of the C5 myotome is graded normal (a grade of 5) and at the C6 myotome greater than or equal to 3, with the sensory level at C3, the motor level is designated as C3. Because there is no C4 myotome to be tested, the sensory level is deferred to, and because the C4 sensory level is not intact, the C4 myotome is also considered not intact. This creates a potential dilemma, because, in this case scenario, if the sensory level were C4 instead of C3, the motor level would have been at C6. This is a 3-level difference from the C3 level and can be very meaningful. If this patient were to gain only 1 sensory level (in this case, the C4 dermatome improving to testing normal), there would be a 3–motor level change (from C3 to C6) even without any muscle grade improvement. Because the motor level is extremely important in designating functional capability appropriately, as well as from a research standpoint, an alternative method for classification may be needed.

Clinical Versus Research Use

The ISNCSCI has been designed for use by clinicians and has been used to document recovery and, as a bedside clinical outcome, examination in a multitude of research studies. The clinical examination as recommended to be performed by the ISNCSCI, allows for classification according to the AIS, but is not, however, a complete neurologic examination. For example, certain important aspects are not included, such as reflexes, and there is no distinction between hyperesthesia and hypoesthesia with the sensory score of "impaired." Furthermore, the AIS only has one designation for persons with a neurologic complete injury (AIS A), but there may be subdivisions needed based on the degree of ZPP sparing, especially if the AIS is used for prognostication. There may also be limitations for research based on the lack of defined motor testing above C5, between T2 and L1, and below S1. The autonomic standards were introduced in 2012 and have added additional ways to document residual function in patients with SCI.[37] ASIA developed an education module on assessing spasticity (Spasticity Assessment Training eLearning Program [SpaSTeP]) in 2013 in an attempt to at least standardize the clinical assessment of spasticity. Looking toward the future, additional modalities may be needed and correlated with the current examination and classification (eg, autonomic, pain, spasticity, or electrophysiological measures) to allow for improved use in research for recovery, medical, and rehabilitation outcomes.

SUMMARY

The goals of the ISNCSCI remain consistent—to have precision and consistency in the definition of neurologic levels and classification of SCI for professionals worldwide in the field to allow for accurate communication. Revisions have been made over the years and many aspects continue to be reviewed by the committee, which has international membership and input. Revisions continue to be considered and changes made based on recommendations and then consensus of the committee.

REFERENCES

1. American Spinal Injury Association. Standards for neurological classification of spinal injury patients. Chicago: ASIA; 1982.
2. Ditunno JF, Graziani V, Tessler A. Neurological assessment in Spinal Cord Injury. Adv Neurol 1997;72:325–33.
3. Michaelis LS. International inquiry on neurological terminology and prognosis in paraplegia and tetraplegia. Paraplegia 1969;7:1–5.
4. Cheshire DJ. A classification of the functional end-results of injury to the cervical spinal cord. Paraplegia 1970;8:70–3.
5. Maroon JC, Alba AA. Classification of acute spinal cord injury, neurological evaluation, and neurosurgical considerations. Crit Care Clin 1987;3:655–77.
6. Allen BL, Ferguson RL, Lehman TR, et al. A mechanistic classification of the lower cervical spine. Spine 1982;7:1–27.
7. Bracken MB, Webb SB, Wagner FC. Classification of the severity of acute spinal cord injury: implications for management. Paraplegia 1978;15:319–26.
8. Roaf R. International classification of spinal injuries. Paraplegia 1972;10:78–84.
9. Chehrazi B, Wagner FC, Collins WF, et al. A scale for evaluation of spinal cord injury. J Neurosurg 1981;54:310–5.
10. Jochheim KA. Problems of classification in traumatic paraplegia and tetraplegia. Paraplegia 1970;8:80–2.
11. Frankel HL, Hancock DO, Hyslop G, et al. The value of postural reduction in initial management of closed injuries of the spine with paraplegia and tetraplegia. Paraplegia 1969;7:179–92.
12. Ditunno JF. American Spinal Injury Standards for Neurological Classification of Spinal Cord Injury: past, present and future. J Am Paraplegia Soc 1993;17:7–11.
13. Tator CH, Rowed DW, Schwartz ML. Sunnybrook cord injury scales for assessing neurological injury and neurological recovery in early management of acute spinal cord injury. In: Tator CH, editor. Early management of acute spinal cord injury. New York: Raven Press; 1982. p. 7–24.
14. Standards for neurological classification of spinal cord injury patients. Chicago: American Spinal Injury Association; 1989.
15. Donovan WH, Wilkerson MA, Rossi D, et al. A test of the ASIA guidelines for classification of spinal cord injury. J Neurol Rehabil 1990;4:39–53.
16. American Spinal Injury Association/International Medical Society of Paraplegia (ASIA/IMSOP). International Standards for Neurological and Functional Classification of Spinal Cord Injury Patients [revised]. Chicago: American Spinal Injury Association; 1992.
17. Waters RL, Adkins RH, Yakura JS. Definition of complete spinal cord injury. Paraplegia 1991;29:573–81.

18. Ditunno JF, Donovan WH, Maynard FM, editors. Reference manual for the international standards for neurological and functional classification of spinal cord injury. Chicago: American Spinal Injury Association (ASIA); 1994.

19. American Spinal Injury Association/International Medical Society of Paraplegia. International Standards for Neurological and Functional Classification of Spinal Cord Injury Patients. Chicago: American Spinal Injury Association; 1996.

20. American Spinal Injury Association/International Medical Society of Paraplegia. International Standards for Neurological Classification of Spinal Cord Injury Patients. Chicago: American Spinal Injury Association; 2000.

21. American Spinal Injury Association. Reference manual for the International Standards for Neurological Classification of Spinal Cord Injury. Chicago: American Spinal Injury Association; 2003.

22. Available at: www.asia-spinalinjury.org/elearning/elearning.php. Accessed May 16, 2014.

23. Waring WP 3rd, Biering-Sorensen F, Burns S, et al. 2009 review and revisions of the international standards for the neurological classification of spinal cord injury. J Spinal Cord Med 2010;33(4):346–52.

24. Kirshblum SC, Burns S, Biering-Sorensen F, et al. International standards for neurological classification of spinal cord injury (Revised 2011). J Spinal Cord Med 2011;34(6):535–46.

25. Kirshblum SC, Waring W, Biering-Sorensen F, et al. Reference for the 2011 revision of the International Standards for Neurological Classification of Spinal Cord Injury. J Spinal Cord Med 2011;34(6):547–54.

26. Vogel LC, Samdani A, Chafetz R, et al. Intra-rater agreement of the anorectal exam and classification of injury severity in children with spinal cord injury. Spinal Cord 2009;47(9):687–91.

27. Schuld C, Wiese J, Franz S, et al, EMSCI Study Group. Effect of formal training in scaling, scoring and classification of the International Standards for Neurological Classification of Spinal Cord Injury. Spinal Cord 2013;51(4):282–8.

28. Hayes KC, Hsieh JT, Wolfe DL, et al. Classifying incomplete spinal cord injury syndromes: algorithms based on the International Standards for Neurological and Functional Classification of Spinal Cord Injury Patients. Arch Phys Med Rehabil 2000;81(5):644–52.

29. Chafetz RS, Prak S, Mulcahey MJ. Computerized Classification of Neurologic Injury Based on the International Standards for Classification of Spinal Cord Injury. J Spinal Cord Med 2009;32(5):532–7.

30. Schuld C, Wiese J, Hug A, et al, Weidner EM-SCI Study Group. Computer implementation of the international standards for neurological classification of spinal cord injury for consistent and efficient derivation of its subscores including handling of data from not testable segments. J Neurotrauma 2012;29(3):453–61.

31. Available at: http://ais.emsci.org. Accessed May 16, 2014.

32. Available at: http://isncscialgorithm.com. Accessed May 16, 2014.

33. Kirshblum SC, Biering-Sorensen F, Betz R. International Standards for Neurological Classification of Spinal Cord Injury: cases with classification challenges. J Spinal Cord Med 2014;37(2):120–7.

34. Pouw MH, van Middlendorp JJ, van Kempen A, et al. Diagnostic criteria of traumatic central cord syndrome. Part 1. A systematic review of clinical descriptors and scores. Spinal Cord 2010;48:652–6.

35. Van Middendorp JJ, Pouw MH, Hayes LC, et al. Diagnostic criteria of traumatic central cord syndrome. Part 2. A questionnaire survey among spine specialists. Spinal Cord 2010;48:657–63.

36. Roth EJ, Park T, Pang T, et al. Traumatic cervical Brown-Sequard and Brown-Sequard plus syndromes: the spectrum of presentations and outcomes. Paraplegia 1991;29:582–9.

37. Krassioukov A, Biering-Sørensen F, Donovan W, et al. International standards to document remaining autonomic function after spinal cord injury. J Spinal Cord Med 2012;35:202–11.

Hypothermia as a Clinical Neuroprotectant

 CrossMark

Andrew L. Sherman, MD, MS[a],*, Michael Y. Wang, MD[b]

KEYWORDS

- Spinal cord injury • Hypothermia • Neuroprotection • ASIA score • Trauma
- Methylprednisolone

KEY POINTS

- Applying hypothermia for the purposes of neuroprotection started nearly 100 years ago, initially used to treat brain abscesses. Applied therapeutic hypothermia has evolved over the years and with modern techniques has become more practical to use.
- Therapeutic hypothermia has been used to provide neuroprotection and minimize tissue injury in several conditions. These conditions include but are not limited to spinal cord injury, traumatic brain injury, stroke, cardiac arrest, burn injury, and subarachnoid hemorrhage.
- Therapeutic hypothermia can help after spinal cord injury at both phases of injury—the primary phase that leads to direct spinal cord tissue damage and the secondary injury phase that leads to apoptosis and further spinal cord damage.
- Initial pilot studies suggest that applying therapeutic hypothermia might lead to improved functional outcome. However, larger multicenter trials are needed to prove these findings.

INTRODUCTION: HISTORY OF HYPOTHERMIA AS A NEUROPROTECTANT

Applying hypothermia for the purposes of neuroprotection, originally termed "hibernation," started nearly 100 years ago. Initially, the treatment was used in patients with intracranial disease from abscess and high fevers, which could lead to severe brain injury.[1] As knowledge regarding neurotrauma has increased and revealed the complex pathophysiology of "secondary neural injury cascades," interest in preventing such secondary damage using hypothermia (and preventing hyperthermia) re-emerged.

More recently, sophisticated cooling systems using thermocouples and feedback sensors have enabled precise and sustained core temperature regulation. These new systems have improved the safety of therapeutic hypothermia (TH) to the point that TH can be applied in a more practical manner. These advances have fueled further interest in hypothermia research, and neuroprotection treatment protocols

[a] Department of Physical medicine and Rehabilitation, University of Miami Miller School of Medicine, 1611 Northwest 12th Avenue, 9th Floor, Miami, FL 33136, USA; [b] Department of Neurological Surgery, University of Miami Miller School of Medicine, 1095 Northwest, 14th Terrace, Miami, FL 33136, USA
* Corresponding author.
E-mail address: asherman@med.miami.edu

Phys Med Rehabil Clin N Am 25 (2014) 519–529
http://dx.doi.org/10.1016/j.pmr.2014.04.003
1047-9651/14/$ – see front matter © 2014 Elsevier Inc. All rights reserved.

have been developed for a wide variety of central nervous system pathologies, such as traumatic brain injury and spinal cord injury (SCI). Finally, with increased interest, new outcome studies have been started and results are being published that support TH as a safe and effective intervention.

The first publication on the use of TH in clinical neuroprotection was a case of traumatic brain injury in 1943. The process was termed "generalized refrigeration."[2] In 1951 and 1956, two additional case reports using TH, now termed "hibernation," on patients with brain abscesses were published.[1,3] Later studies focused on development of animal models and the idea that TH could reduce secondary damage after brain trauma by reducing cerebral ischemia.[4] This idea was paramount in a study published in 1996 looking prospectively at effects of moderate hypothermia (core temperature 32.5°C–33.0°C for 24 hrs.) in 10 patients with severe closed head injury (Glasgow Coma Scale score <7).[5] Seven of these patients made a good recovery. The effects seen were reductions in intracranial hypertension, cerebral oxygen consumption, and cerebral ischemia. Another study looked at 46 patients subjected to TH versus standardized treatment. They found the cooling group had reduced seizures and more patients recovering to a good recovery/moderate disability level versus remaining at a severe disability/vegetative/dead level.[6]

However, concerns were also raised in these studies regarding potential hazards of the TH treatment. Although reversible with rewarming, increased levels of lipase and amylase were seen. Although a statistically significant increase in the partial tromboplastin time and prothrombin time, just out of the normal range, was found during and after rewarming, there were no clinically significant problems with bleeding. Increased rates of sepsis were not clinically significant.[5]

CORE TEMPERATURE REGULATION AND HYPOTHERMIA

TH is defined simply as the reduction of mean body core temperature to create some medical benefit. As warm-blooded mammals, humans regulate their core body temperature within a constant and narrow range and will not tolerate even short periods of hypothermia without engaging compensatory mechanisms. Hypothermia induces a variety of human responses to combat the hypothermia. These thermoregulatory mechanisms in humans have 2 components: behavioral and hypothalamic.[7] External behavioral mechanisms to increase core temperature could include clothing, shelter, warm baths, or seeking environments with higher external temperature. In the intensive care unit (ICU) setting, patients often have no or limited control over these mechanisms.

Internal mechanisms of reducing hypothermia include arteriovenous shunting, inducted vasoconstriction, and shivering. The site of internal thermoregulation is considered to be the hypothalamus.[8] Shivering is involuntary and creates muscle activity that increases metabolic heat production. In general, as the temperature drops less than 36.5°C, shivering begins. Shivering is initiated by regional vasoconstriction and becomes severe at core temperatures under 35.5°C. Nonshivering thermogenesis does occur in adults to combat hypothermia but plays a minor role compared with shivering.[9] Shivering is a highly effective mechanism that increases metabolic heat production many times over, thus effectively raising core body temperature. Therefore, in any type of TH treatment, these compensatory mechanisms need to be curtailed, monitored, or modified.

MECHANISM OF NEUROPROTECTION IN HYPOTHERMIA
Metabolic Rate of Oxygen Consumed

The primary neuroprotective effect of hypothermia applied as therapy in acute neurotrauma is a reduction in the metabolic rate of oxygen consumed by the brain and spinal cord. By reducing the metabolic rate of oxygen consumption, the energy rate used might be reduced and glucose utilization might be improved.[10] One measure of brain oxygen consumption places the magnitude of the reduction at 5% for each degree Celsius the body temperature is reduced.[7]

Additionally, neurotrauma often causes a hypermetabolic state because the damaged neuronal tissue deals with repair and inflammatory mediators and free radicals that need to be "cleaned up." As a result, lactate accumulates and alters pH, creating an acidotic state. Applied hypothermia, by slowing metabolism, has been thought to reduce interstitial lactate accumulation. For every degree (Celsius) that body temperature decreases, the pH increases by 0.016.[11] Therefore, one theory is that TH protects from neurologic injury by reducing acidosis. Despite the "neatness" of this theory, other investigators have questioned the actual measurements and theory altogether.[4]

CLINICAL APPLICATION
Patient Evaluation Overview

The patients who are felt to be candidates for TH share certain aspects of their neurologic pathophysiology. The main unifying theme is that all patients have conditions exacerbated by secondary injury to the central nervous system. The mechanisms of such secondary injury include the following: Wallerian degeneration, vascular ischemia, ionic alterations, accumulation of neurotransmitters in a pathologic fashion, release of arachidonic acid and production of free radicals, formation of cytotoxic edema, hyperinflammatory response, and failure of adenosine triposphate–dependent processes. The protective effects of hypothermia are multimodal, involving suppression of the injury-induced immune response and inflammation[12,13] reductions in vasogenic edema, inhibited polymorphonuclear chemotaxis,[14,15] and reductions in gliosis.[16] Hypothermia also reduces glutamate-mediated neurotoxicity and oxygen-free radical production.[17,18] The classic conditions where these processes occur is traumatic brain injury and SCI; thus, these are 2 key problem areas where TH has been used to prevent secondary neuronal damage. Similarly, patients post-acute ischemic stroke and hemorrhagic stroke also fit the profile of those who could stand to benefit from TH.

In the setting of neurotrauma, when a new intervention is proposed, complete neurologic recovery is typically the main goal. However, with even small or incremental gains, these patients can often see tremendous functional improvements. For cervical SCI patients, incremental recovery of just one spinal level can translate into meaningful gains in the ability to perform self-care and functional tasks. For example, improving from a C6 SCI level to a C7 injury level can translate into the ability to propel a manual wheelchair or manipulate a urinary catheter. Improvement to a C8 level increases hand function to the point that an assistive device may not be needed. Therefore, interventions that allow even incremental neurologic improvement are important in this group of patients.

Another group where TH is being explored is in those with aneurysmal subarachnoid hemorrhage (SAH).[19] TH has been used to treat the development of delayed cerebral ischemia, which can progress to cerebral infarction associated with poor outcomes. The focus of hypothermia treatment has been to reduce cerebral vasospasm, which is a delayed morphologic narrowing of cerebral arteries, occurring 4 to 10 days after SAH. TH has also been considered for patients with SAH during aneurysm surgery[20] and immediately after rupture at initial presentation.

Cooling methodologies
The development of closed circuit intravascular cooling catheters has greatly enhanced the safety and efficacy of hypothermia delivery. External cooling through

transcutaneous pads or suits can provide a noninvasive method for reducing body temperature, but precise control remains elusive and surface heat exchange devices can interfere with sensory neurologic testing (**Fig. 1**).

Two brands of Food and Drug Administration (FDA)-approved catheters have become commercially available using closed-circuit feedback mechanisms to regulate heat exchange. Thus, these devices not only increase the rate at which core body temperature is reduced, but also effectively regulate the temperature within a narrow therapeutic window. Because skin sensation contributes disproportionately to the perception and discomfort of cooling, endovascular cooling is also far more comfortable for awake patients than is surface cooling. Skin counterwarming can even be used with endovascular cooling to lower the shiver threshold and improve comfort without adversely affecting the core temperature.

Bradycardia is a predictable consequence of cooling, with a mean decrease in 10 to 12 beats per minute when comparing baseline to target temperature. Intravenous adrenergic agents, which are frequently used to treat hypotension from neurogenic shock, can also be helpful for treating bradycardia. External pacing for excessive rate depression in refractory cases can be used temporarily as well.

Shivering has also been associated with systemic cooling. In addition to patient discomfort, shivering increases metabolic demands and can lead to difficulties in reaching target body temperature. For patients who are not on mechanical ventilation, the management of shivering can typically be accomplished with the use of pharmacologic agents. In a review by Kranke, meperidine, 25 mg was found to be an effective agent for control of acute symptoms.[21] Control of shivering will be at the discretion of the treating center, but because of its adverse effects on patient comfort and effects on body temperature, it should be pharmacologically treated. Shivering is more common following thoracic level injuries and is less commonly encountered with tetraplegic patients.

HYPOTHERMIA IN THE SCI POPULATION
Historical Perspective

For the past 7 decades, TH has been applied in the setting of SCI.[22] The idea of using TH in SCI was brought forth in the 1950s in a dog model and in 1968 in a study on primates.[23,24] Localized spinal cord cooling with a simple liquid perfusion unit produced effective selective reduction of spinal cord temperature. Thirteen monkeys that had complete lower extremity paraplegia following induced impact injury at T10 followed by incision of the dura 4 hours later and localized spinal cord cooling for 3 more hours showed an excellent return of neurologic function. Studies like these led to increased interest in cooling the spinal cord locally in humans rather than systemically, as for brain injury or stroke. In addition, local application of cooling in SCI was possible for short periods of time as most patients with traumatic SCI had to undergo surgery with direct exposure of the injured segment of spinal cord.

Despite this early interest, enthusiasm for TH for treatment of SCI waned in the 1970s and 1980s due to the emerging availability of new pharmacologic agents for neuroprotection. Initial study results created great excitement in the use of high-dose methylprednisolone, which for a period of time became standard care for acute SCI.[25–28] Other antiinflammatory pharmacologic agents such as naloxone and tirilazad mesylate also showed initial promise but ultimately proved ineffective. By the mid 1990s, doubt emerged regarding the use of methylprednisolone.[29] Further analysis of the original published research suggested a higher rate of complications and the amount of neurologic recovery was felt to be minimal,[30] and ultimately high-dose methylprednisolone for SCI was abandoned in most trauma centers.

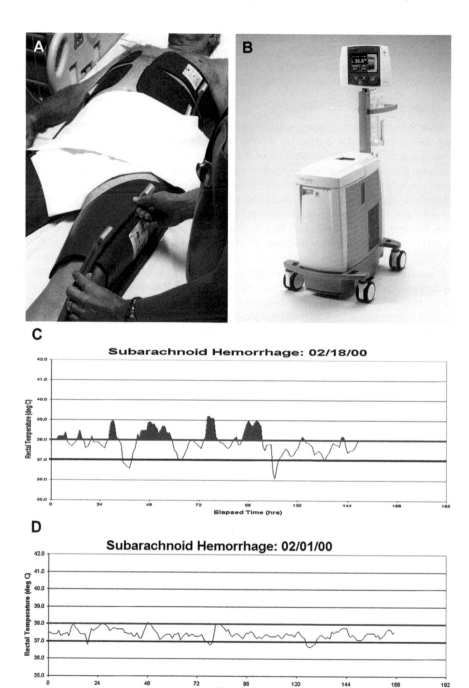

Fig. 1. (*A*) Surface cooling using adhesive heat exchange pads with cooling fluid circulated through them. (*B*) Intravascular cooling console with heat exchange catheter placed through the femoral vein. (*C, D*) The console regulates temperature via a feedback mechanism, resulting in improvements in tight temperature control. ([*B*] *Courtesy of* ZOLL, Chelmsford, MA; with permission.)

Because currently there are no proved effective neuroprotectants for acute SCI, hypothermia is being investigated as a potential low-risk intervention for treating this patient population where incremental improvements in long-term neurologic function can have a significant health-related and socioeconomic impact.

Contemporary Animal SCI Studies

Numerous animal studies using various models of mechanical SCI in diverse species have demonstrated the protective effects of hypothermia. Dimar and colleagues[31] investigated direct *in vivo* incubation of the rat thoracic spinal cord in isotonic baths of varying temperatures. When normothermic environments were compared with local cooling to 19°C, improved clinical outcomes as measured by the Basso, Beattie, and Bresnahan (BBB) score were demonstrated in the cooled group when spacer compression of the spinal cord was applied. This treatment effect was not robust when the same model was used to test the effects of spinal cord contusions using the NYU impactor or with a combination of contusion and spacer compression.[31]

In 1992, Martinez-Arizala and Green at the University of Miami reported that pre and post-treatment with moderate hypothermia (31°C–32°C) was effective in decreasing the degree of hemorrhage at the site of primary injury.[12] This study provided evidence that an early cooling strategy might lessen the deleterious effects of trauma on the spinal cord microvasculature and reduce local swelling and also confirmed that deeper cooling may not be necessary to realize hypothermia's neuroprotective effects.

Follow-up preclinical studies by Yu and colleagues[13] have demonstrated that systemic hypothermia resulted in concomitant epidural cooling that was neuroprotective for contusive injuries. Rats exposed to surface cooling with a target temperature of 32°C to 33°C were compared with normothermic rats following a T10 spinal cord contusion with an NYU impactor (10 g weight with 12.5 mm drop). Hypothermia was instituted 30 minutes after SCI and maintained for 4 hours. Monitoring of systemic (rectal) temperature showed close correlation with the temperature in the epidural space.[13] Open field locomotor BBB testing demonstrated that rats exposed to hypothermia exhibited improved scores as early as 1 week following injury. Furthermore, this trend continued throughout the study and was more significant at the end of the 44 days studied. Final BBB scores averaged 13.3 ± 0.47 in the hypothermia-treated animals versus 10.8 ± 0.44 in normothermic animals ($P = .0024$).[13]

Histologic analysis of the contused spinal cord at 7 and 44 days post-injury demonstrated the hemorrhagic necrosis, cell loss, axonal swelling, and vacuolization typically seen following SCI. However, in the hypothermia-treated group, sparing of gray and white matter was seen with smaller associated contusion volumes and reduced rostral-caudal spread. Volumetric assessments of the area of contusion size were obtained by sectioning 16 mm of spinal cord around the T10 impact site. Sixteen representative 10 μm thick slices were then analyzed histopathologically using hematoxylin and eosin staining. This analysis demonstrated a mean 15.8% reduction in lesion size in the hypothermia-treated animals ($P = .01$) (**Fig. 2**).

These findings in a thoracic model of rodent SCI have been confirmed using a recently developed rat model for cervical SCI at the University of Miami. Using the methodology as described by Pearse and colleagues,[32] a C5 contusion injury was created with the Ohio State electromagnetic SCI device, delivering a 3 Kdyn impact and displacing the neural tissues 0.95 mm. Rats randomized to receive moderate hypothermia at 33°C delivered externally for 2 hours after injury were found to have improved neurologic outcomes in forelimb function. Measures of forelimb gripping force were reduced from 1.15 ± 0.10 Nm in normal animals to 0.42 ± 0.10 Nm (64% reduction) in normothermic versus 0.56 ± 0.07 Nm (51% reduction) in

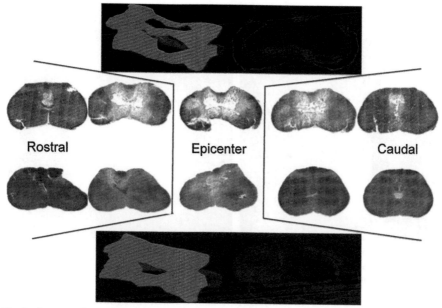

Fig. 2. Cross-sections of rat spinal cord H&E stained following experimental traumatic injury. Normothermic animals. The spinal cord with therapeutic hypothermia. Note the reduced cell loss cranially and caudally distant from the injury in cooled animals.

hypothermic animals (P<.05).[33] The weight-supported forelimb hanging test improved this ability from 3.3 ± 1.1 seconds to 5.8 ± 1.0 seconds (P<.01).[34]

Preliminary Clinical Evidence of Efficacy—Evaluation of Outcome and Long-term Recommendations

A pilot study to assess the safety and effects of moderate intravascular hypothermia (33.0°C ± 0.5°C) in the setting of acute traumatic cervical SCI was recently published.[35] The study protocol by Levi and colleagues included tetraplegic patients aged 16 to 65 years with complete (AIS Grade A) loss of neurologic function with consent obtained and a goal of initiation of cooling within 6 hours of injury (University of Miami IRB approved protocol # 20071018). Exclusion criteria included penetrating injuries; hyperthermia on admission; severe systemic injury or bleeding; blood dyscrasias; history of coagulopathy, arrhythmia, or severe cardiac disease; pregnancy; pancreatitis; Raynaud syndrome; cord transection; patients who are intubated and sedated before initial examination; and patients showing neurologic improvement within 12 hours of injury (**Fig. 3**). Reasons for the exclusion criteria was to attempt to isolate patients with functional and neurologic deficits that were due only to the SCI to best attempt to see the effect of a single variable—the hypothermia. Additionally, some of the conditions excluded were excluded because they do not allow for an "accurate enough" prehypothermia neurologic examination.

Patients were cooled intravascularly with a target temperature of 33.0°C per hour at a maximum rate of 0.5°C per hour, with maintenance of hypothermia for 48 hours using the Alsius CoolGard Icy Catheter (Zoll Medical, Chelmsford, Massachusetts), an FDA-approved (510k #K030421) cooling catheter placed into the femoral vein. This cooling was followed by slow rewarming at 0.1°C per hour to prevent rebound hyperthermia.[35] Catheter placement occurred in the Emergency Department and patients

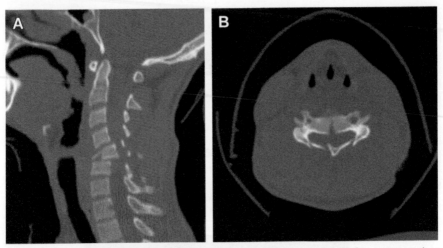

Fig. 3. Case example of a patient treated with therapeutic hypothermia for a C5 tear drop fracture with AIS Grade A SCI after falling out of a tree. (*A*) Sagittal and (*B*) axial computed tomographic scan views of the fracture.

were managed in the ICU while hypothermic. There was no contraindication to early surgery, traction, or imaging. Blood pressure support was used, as needed, to maintain a mean arterial pressure of more than 90 mm Hg. A second confirmatory neurologic examination was performed 12 hours after injury with no sedation. Over a period of 25 months, 14 eligible patients were enrolled into the treatment.[35]

Mean time injury to initiation of hypothermia was 7.40 ± 0.27 hours, and time from initiation to target temperature was 2.72 ± 0.42 hours. Cooling to target temperature was achieved in all patients with a mean rate of 0.83°C/h (SD = 0.43). All patients

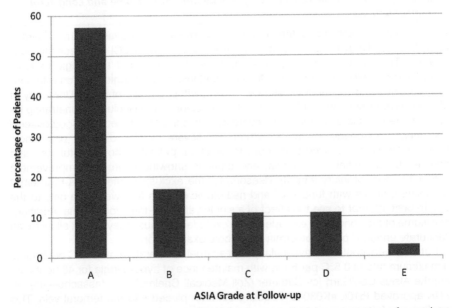

Fig. 4. Conversion of AIS Grade A SCI patients from an initial presentation of complete quadriplegia.

underwent cervical traction and surgery for decompression and stabilization, with 10 patients (71.4%) having surgery within 24 hours of injury. None of the patients received high-dose Solu-Medrol.

The distribution of injuries included C4 (21.4%), C5 (50%), and C6 (28.6%). There were no instances of neurologic worsening, and there were no early conversions from completeness of injury, with all patients motor and sensory complete at 12 hours post-injury. At the last follow-up (median 52 weeks), 6 of the 14 patients (42.8%) converted from AIS A to an incomplete SCI. Three (21.4%) regained sensory function, converting to AIS B, and 3 regained motor function converting to AIS C (14.3%) or D (7.1%) (**Fig. 4**). The remainder remained neurologically complete at early (2-week) follow-up. All recoveries occurred following discharge from their acute hospitalization.

SUMMARY

It is clear from published case reports, pilot studies, and animal data that the use of TH in the setting of acute deserves further study. Could TH become the standard intervention in all acute episodes of SCI? Only time and the outcome of future studies will tell. However, the potential promise of preservation or even return of lost neurologic function after acute SCI through the use of TH is intriguing and exciting. Therefore, the authors support the initiation of future studies preferably via a multicenter format where larger numbers of patients receiving the TH can be reviewed.

REFERENCES

1. Babe J, Delgado. Otogenous cerebral abscess treated by surgical intervention and hibernation. Acta Otorinolaryngol Iber Am 1956;7:212–20 [in Spanish].
2. Henderson AR. Temple Fay MD, Uncomfortable Crusader and Harbinger of Human refrigeration, 1895-1963. J Neurosurg 1963;20:627–34.
3. Zdravev P. Treatment of cerebral hernia following surgery of an otogenous brain abscess. Ann Otolaryngol 1951;68:201–5.
4. Busto R, Dietrich WD, Globus MY, et al. The importance of brain temperature in cerebral ischemic injury. Stroke 1989;20:1113–4.
5. Metz C, Holzschuh M, Bein T, et al. Moderate hypothermia in patients with severe head injury: cerebral and extracerebral effects. J Neurosurg 1996;85:533–41.
6. Clifton GL, Allen S, Barrodale P, et al. A phase II study of moderate hypothermia in severe brain injury. J Neurotrauma 1993;10:263–71 [discussion: 273].
7. Faridar A, Bershad EM, Emiru T, et al. Therapeutic hypothermia in stroke and traumatic brain injury. Front Neurol 2011;2:80.
8. Sessler DI. Temperature monitoring and perioperative thermoregulation. Anesthesiology 2008;109:318–38.
9. Jessen K. An assessment of human regulatory nonshivering thermogenesis. Acta Anaesthesiol Scand 1980;24:138–43.
10. Yenari M, Wijman C, Steinberg G. Effects of hypothermia on cerebral metabolism, blood flow, and autoregulation. In: Mayer S, Sessler D, editors. Therapeutic hypothermia. New York: Marcel Dekker; 2008. p. 141–78.
11. Varon J, Acosta P. Therapeutic hypothermia: past, present, and future. Chest 2008;133:1267–74.
12. Martinez-Arizala A, Green B. Hypothermia in spinal cord injury. J Neurotrauma 1992;9:S497–505.
13. Yu C, Jimenez O, Marcillo A, et al. Beneficial effects of modest systemic hypothermia on locomotor function and histopathological damage following contusion-induced spinal cord injury in rats. J Neurosurg 2000;93:85–93.

14. Bernard SA, Mac CJ, Buist M. Experience with prolonged induced hypothermia in severe head injury. Crit Care 1999;3:167–72.
15. Chatzipantelli K, Yanagawa Y, Marcillo A, et al. Posttraumatic hypothermia reduces polymorphonuclear leukocyte accumulation following spinal cord injury in rats. J Neurotrauma 2000;17:321–32.
16. Westergren H, Farooque M, Olsson Y, et al. Motor function changes in the rat following severe spinal cord injury. Does treatment with moderate systemic hypothermia improve functional outcome? Acta Neurochir (Wien) 2000;142:567–73.
17. Marsala M, Sorkin L, Yaksh T. Transient spinal ischemia in rat: characterization of spinal cord blood flow, extracellular amino acid release, and concurrent histopathological damage. J Cereb Blood Flow Metab 1994;14:604–14.
18. Sunde K, Pytte M, Jacobsen D, et al. Implementation of a standardised treatment protocol for post resuscitation care after out-of-hospital cardiac arrest. Resuscitation 2007;73:29–39.
19. Seule M, Muroi C, Sikorski C, et al. Therapeutic hypothermia reduces middle cerebral artery flow velocity in patients with severe aneurysmal subarachnoid hemorrhage. Neurocritical Care 2014;20(2):255–62.
20. Todd MM, Hindman BJ, Clarke WR, et al. Mild intraoperative hypothermia during surgery for intracranial aneurysm. N Engl J Med 2005;352:135–45.
21. Kranke P, Eberhart L, Roewer N, et al. Pharmacologic treatment of postoperative shivering: a quantitative systematic review of randomized controlled trials. Anesth Analg 2002;94:453–60.
22. Cappuccino A, Bisson L, Carpenter B, et al. The use of systemic hypothermia for the treatment of an acute cervical spinal cord injury in a professional football player. Spine 2010;35:E57–62.
23. Albin M, White R, Acosta-Rica G, et al. Study of functional recovery produced by delayed localized cooling of spinal cord injury in primates. J Neurosurg 1968;29:113–20.
24. Albin M, White R, Yashon D, et al. Effects of cooling on spinal cord trauma. J Trauma 1969;9:1000–8.
25. Bracken MB, Shepard MJ, Collins WF, et al. A randomized, controlled trial of methylprednisolone or naloxone in the treatment of acute spinal-cord injury. Results of the Second National Acute Spinal Cord Injury Study. N Engl J Med 1990;322:1405–11.
26. Bracken MB, Shepard MJ, Collins WF Jr, et al. Methylprednisolone or naloxone treatment after acute spinal cord injury: 1-year follow-up data. Results of the second National Acute Spinal Cord Injury Study. J Neurosurg 1992;76:23–31.
27. Bracken MB, Shepard MJ, Hellenbrand KG, et al. Methylprednisolone and neurological function 1 year after spinal cord injury. Results of the National Acute Spinal Cord Injury Study. J Neurosurg 1985;63:704–13.
28. Bracken MB, Shepard MJ, Holford TR, et al. Administration of methylprednisolone for 24 or 48 hours or tirilazad mesylate for 48 hours in the treatment of acute spinal cord injury. Results of the Third National Acute Spinal Cord Injury Randomized Controlled Trial. National Acute Spinal Cord Injury Study. JAMA 1997;277:1597–604.
29. Hurlbert R. The role of steroids in acute spinal cord injury: an evidence-based analysis. Spine 2001;26:S55.
30. Hugenholtz H, Cass DE, Dvorak MF, et al. High-dose methylprednisolone for acute closed spinal cord injury–only a treatment option. Can J Neurol Sci 2002;29:227–35.
31. Dimar J, Shields C, Zhang Y, et al. The role of directly applied hypothermia in spinal cord injury. Spine 2000;25:2294–302.

32. Pearse D, Lo T, Cho K, et al. Histopathological and behavioral characterization of a novel cervical spinal cord displacement contusion in the rat. Neurotrauma 2005;22:680–702.
33. Meyer O, Tilson H, Byrd W, et al. A method for the routine assessment of fore- and hindlimb strength of rats and mice. Neurobehav Toxicol 1979;1:233–6.
34. Diener P, Bregman B. Fetal spinal cord transplants support the development of target reaching and coordinated postural adjustments after neonatal spinal cord injury. J Neurosci 1998;18:763–78.
35. Levi A, Green B, Wang M, et al. Clinical application of modest hypothermia after spinal cord injury. J Neurotrauma 2008;26:407–15.

Assessment of Neuromuscular Conditions Using Ultrasound

Robert W. Irwin, MD[a,b,*], Erin T. Wolff, MD[a]

KEYWORDS

- Ultrasound • Shoulder • Elbow • Wrist • Nerve • Tendon • Elastography

KEY POINTS

- Pain is commonly reported in persons with spinal cord injury.
- Ultrasound is inexpensive, portable, and accessible.
- Ultrasound has been shown to be a useful imaging modality for nerve, muscle, and tendons in the able-bodied population.
- Ultrasound has been used to assess for changes in the spinal cord–injured population before and after exercise so that early changes can be found and intervention can be preventative.
- Newer measures, including elastography, have the potential to facilitate diagnosis and allow earlier detection of pathology.

INTRODUCTION

No two spinal cord injuries are exactly the same.[1–29] Not only are there significant differences in those with cervical, thoracic, and lumbar injuries, and complete and incomplete injuries, but there are many individual differences in patients with the same type of injury. Persons with a spinal cord injury (SCI) have reported various musculoskeletal pains that can occur early on or more remotely from the injury. The frequency and risk of certain types of musculoskeletal pain are increased in certain injury levels; up to 73% of persons with an SCI may suffer some form of musculoskeletal pain during their lifetime.[30] Most of the musculoskeletal injuries suffered are non-traumatic in origin, and a result of poor posture and overuse.[30] Therefore, most of

Funding Sources: National Institute on Disability and Rehabilitation Research/U.S. Department of Energy grant # H133N110003 (R.W. Irwin); None (E.T. Wolff).
Conflict of Interest: None.
[a] Department of Rehabilitation Medicine, Miller School of Medicine, University of Miami, 1120 North West 14th Street, Miami, FL 33136, USA; [b] Medical Education, Miller School of Medicine, University of Miami, 1120 North West 14th Street, Miami, FL 33136, USA
* Corresponding author. Department of Rehabilitation Medicine, Miller School of Medicine, University of Miami, Miami, FL.
E-mail address: rirwin@med.miami.edu

Phys Med Rehabil Clin N Am 25 (2014) 531–543
http://dx.doi.org/10.1016/j.pmr.2014.04.009
1047-9651/14/$ – see front matter © 2014 Elsevier Inc. All rights reserved.

these injuries and pain syndromes can be treated medically through rehabilitation, and may even be prevented through education on proper body mechanics, posture, and simple balancing exercises. Here, we outline the scope of the problem, and discuss how, with improvements in technology, ultrasound (US) is changing the way we assess these complaints. We also will address some of the newer data on differences in musculoskeletal structures that can be seen in anatomic structures in the SCI population when compared with the able-bodied population.

NATURE OF THE PROBLEM

After SCI, the upper extremities (UEs) are often called on to become weight-bearing limbs. This is seen in those who now need to use their arms for transfers, positioning, pressure reliefs, and locomotion. The increased use of the UEs in wheelchair propulsion, transfers, and activities of daily living is believed to increase the incidence of injury to the shoulders, elbows, and wrists.[31] The structures involved include tendons/ligaments, nerves, and joints. Although some of these issues may be acute and short lived, many often progress to chronic problems. In patients with SCI, 69% to 76% report pain in the UEs, most often the shoulders.[32] The incidence of pain in the UE has been well characterized and shows the following:

- Shoulder pain ranges between 30% and 73%[32–36]
- Elbow pain is approximately 32%[37]
- Wrist and hand pain ranges between 30% and 64%[33,35,38,39]

This is most likely the result of the inability of the person with SCI to rest the affected structure because he or she is now more dependent on the UEs. Chronic injuries can be a significant source of increased disability in this population. Treatments may require time and even surgery. These chronic injuries can interfere with mobility and transfers. As a result, it is important to address these issues as soon as possible.

POSSIBLE AFFECTED STRUCTURES
Muscles/Tendons and Joints

Overuse of tendons and ligaments is one of the major issues when the UE becomes a weight-bearing structure. The sheer and effects of gravity can affect multiple structures. These in turn can affect the bones and joints. These overuse musculoskeletal injuries carry a significant morbidity in this population. Any structure in the UE has the potential of being injured with the new demands of transfers, wheelchair propulsion, and pressure releases. These structures may be only mildly injured, as in tendinitis or strains, or more seriously damaged, as in a tear. Although many of these injuries may be self-limited in able-bodied persons, this is less likely the case, as it is more difficult to rest the injured area in the SCI population and an acute tendinitis can develop into a chronic tendinosis. A list of the muscles and tendons commonly affected is seen in **Box 1**.

Nerves

Although we see a significant number of musculoskeletal injuries as mentioned previously, neurologic injuries also play a role in contributing to pain in persons with SCI. These injuries may be difficult to diagnose as a result of their symptoms. Many persons with SCI have residual numbness and tingling, which is a common symptom of early peripheral nerve disease and may, therefore, mask the development of peripheral nerve problems. For instance, persons with C6 or C7 tetraplegia may have hand numbness and tingling at the level of injury, which may mask the early symptoms of

Box 1
Structures susceptible to overuse injuries
Shoulder:
Rotator cuff tendons
Biceps tendon
Glenohumeral joint
Acromioclavicular joint
Subacromial bursa
Glenohumeral labrum
Elbow:
Lateral epicondyle
Medial epicondyle
Olecranon bursa
Wrist/Hand:
Wrist flexors
Wrist extensors
Carpal metacarpal joint
Extensor/Abductor pollicis

either carpal tunnel syndrome or ulnar neuropathy at the elbow. Not only are entrapments possible, but, with the increase in diabetes in the population in general, the SCI population is also at risk for diabetic peripheral neuropathy. Sites and nerves that may be entrapped or injured in the distal upper extremities include the following:

- Median nerve
    Carpal tunnel syndrome
    Pronator syndrome
- Ulnar nerve
    Entrapment at the Guyon canal
    Ulnar nerve entrapment at the elbow
- Radial nerve
- Other peripheral nerves

ULTRASOUND
Why Use Ultrasound?

One of the issues in the past in assessing pain in SCI is the ability to assess the structure and find the cause of the pain. Although bones may be easily assessed with radiographs, soft tissue injuries require a different modality. Oftentimes, magnetic resonance imaging (MRI) or computerized tomography scans are used. These come with significant costs and need to be scheduled. Over the past decade, with the advent of improved technology, US has started to make the move from the radiology suite to the clinic setting in the form of portable US machines. This modality now allows instant assessment of the structures in question and can help guide treatments. Higher-frequency transducers have allowed for better characterization of tendons and nerves, especially in the more shallow structures as seen in the shoulder, elbow, and wrist. **Table 1** illustrates the relative cost and advantages of the major imaging modalities.

Table 1
The relationship of cost, accessibility, structures assessed, and advantages of the major imaging modalities

Diagnostic Modality	Structures Visualized	Cost	Accessibility	Advantage/ Disadvantage
MRI	All structures	$$$	Within a week usually	• Cannot use with pacemaker/defibrillator • Often cannot use with loose metal fragments • Hard to use in claustrophobia
CT scan	Bones and some soft tissues	$$	Within a week usually	• Can use with pacemaker/ defibrillators • Poor soft tissue visualization
US	Tendons, ligaments and nerves	$	In the clinic	• Can use with pacemaker/ defibrillators • Portable
Radiograph	Bone and joints	$	Day of clinic visit	• Does not show soft tissue

Abbreviations: CT, computed tomography; MRI, magnetic resonance imaging; US, ultrasound; $, inexpensive; $$, moderately expensive; $$$, expensive.

STUDIES EVALUATING STRUCTURES USING US IN THE SCI POPULATION

To date, the studies evaluating tendons and nerves in the SCI population have been few. Some of the studies have been undertaken solely to characterize the tendon structure and develop a quantitative measurement for these structures.[12,27,40] The questions that remain to be answered are the following:

- Are there differences in the nerves and tendons of SCI and able-bodied persons?
- How are tendons and nerves affected by use?
- Is there a difference in the response to use between SCI and able-bodied persons?
- Can we identify those at risk and intervene before there is significant morbidity?

We discuss what has been done in this population and then discuss where the health care industry might be able to maximize the potential of US in this population. There are several studies on US assessment of tendons and nerves in the upper extremities. These studies have focused on the changes that are associated with use in this population.

Study of the Nerves in the SCI Population

In a study comparing sedentary versus wheelchair racers in SCI, the authors found that the racers had fewer nerve injuries overall compared with sedentary wheelchair users; these subjects were assessed with electrodiagnostic testing and not US and suggested that the overall incidence of injuries was low: 3.2% in racers, and 13.6% in sedentary SCI.[41] This is in contrast to the lifetime incidence mentioned earlier in this article. A more recent article found that asymptomatic median neuropathy may even be as high as 25.5% in the paraplegic population.[42] Still, many other studies have found the prevalence of carpal tunnel syndrome to be between 49% and 73%, and that the prevalence increases with the time elapsed from initial injury.[38,40,43–47]

With this information, researchers have begun to evaluate the median nerve's reaction to exercise. In one study by Altinok and colleagues,[1] there was an increase in the cross-sectional area (CSA) of the median nerve at the level of the pisiform, but not at the distal radius in those patients with carpal tunnel syndrome (CTS) than in those without, at baseline, before activities. The study also found that differences between the groups were magnified and showed up in other parameters after provocative exercises imitating work-related stresses. Massy-Westropp and colleagues[48] evaluated normal median nerves with exercise and found an increase in CSA after exercise that returned to baseline in 10 minutes. In 2009, Impink and colleagues[40] evaluated the median nerve of paraplegic patients and the response to exercise and found that the nerve responded differently to exercise in those who had symptoms of CTS compared with those who did not have any symptoms. It is therefore likely that these nerves are different at baseline and with short bouts of exercise, but it is not clear what chronic use changes may be seen in this population.

This information may suggest that researchers should start to evaluate the changes in nerves as a result of exercise, not only in those with symptoms, but also to compare those who use manual wheel chairs with able-bodied controls to see if the nerves respond differently over time in a longitudinal study. This might lead to the ability to identify those at risk for future development of nerve injuries after SCI. It also may be important, once the problems are characterized, to develop an intervention that may prevent or reverse the anatomic changes seen on US.

Tendons in the SCI Population

Tendons may change after SCI and the resultant demands placed on them. To understand these changes, it is helpful to understand what adaptations the tendon makes after an SCI. One study in 2006[49] evaluated tendons below the level of injury in paraplegic patients and able-bodied controls. The findings suggested a decrease in the tendon CSA of the patellar tendon compared with controls. In this study, the tendons of the paraplegic subject underwent electrical stimulation, whereas the able-bodied controls continued their regular recreational activity levels.

There have been several studies attempting to quantitate tendons after exercise. In a study by van Drongelen and colleagues,[27] the biceps tendon CSA and echogenicity were measured before and after a sporting event. They found the echogenicity of the tendon decreased and the size increased. They also found this was directly related to playing time. In one study assessing reliability, they found that the use of one operator was fairly good, but interrater reliability was lacking. They also found that US did not demonstrate changes in tendons, only muscles, after electrical stimulation of lower extremity muscles.[50] Brushoj and colleagues[8] noted that although the CSA may be fairly consistent, the tendon thickness and the thickness measurements were not as reliable.

Another group found the presence of edema in persons with tetraplegia and paraplegia when compared with the able-bodied population.[51] In an attempt to help standardize assessment of tendons in the SCI population, Brose and colleagues[52] developed the US Pathology Rating Scale (USPRS) to quantitate shoulder pathology, and found the changes in the USPRS were related to age, duration of SCI, and weight. Some researchers have advocated a more quantitative set of measures for assessing tendons, but again, the interrater reliability was less than desirable.[12]

The potential future of US in the SCI population

US in the person with SCI has the potential to catch issues early, and allow for adjustment of biomechanics to prevent increased disability. The fact that US machines are becoming more powerful as well as more portable, will allow this tool to be used often and with ease. A patient admitted to the hospital with a new SCI, once stabilized, may then have complaints of shoulder pain, and bedside US may be able to identify a rotator cuff tear or subacromial bursitis, which may interfere with the rehabilitation. This will be a huge advantage, once adopted as standard, to decrease the cost of care in several ways. First, there will be the cost of obtaining an MRI; second, the loss of time to diagnosis (as MRIs may take several days to be performed); and third, treatment on the injury may start earlier, potentially leading to an earlier discharge. At this point in time, the advantages of US in the SCI population have not become common in practice because of several factors. Some of these include that until recently the radiologists have been the only ones able to perform these diagnostic procedures. There are multiple specialty societies who are now offering training for their physicians that in turn will increase the number of those who can perform the procedure. The next step is for standardization of training among different specialties and for the insurance industry to start covering the cost of this when performed by someone other than a radiologist. In addition, the cost of the US machine can still be considerable, and, in the era of cost containment, it may take a while to increase the availability of the US machine in the clinic.

DIAGNOSTIC ULTRASOUND

Although the incidence of injury may be higher in the SCI population, the soft tissue evaluation with US is the same as for able-bodied persons. Consensus statements conclude that musculoskeletal US is for detecting joint synovitis, effusions, fluid collections, and evaluating tendon, muscle, and ligament, but is poor at detecting loose bodies.[53] Jamadar and colleagues[54] found that protocols detected nearly all symptomatic abnormalities in the extremities. Only 2.2% of findings from focal examinations were missed by a protocol-based approach. However, focal examination was more likely to detect abnormalities only in distal joints. They recommended combining protocol and focal examinations. Protocols have been developed for consistent evaluation of the UEs,[54,55] with published descriptions of these evaluations.[5,56]

US STUDIES OF THE SHOULDER IN ABLE-BODIED SUBJECTS

Beggs[5] describes the diagnostic shoulder examination in an article from 2011. The protocol can be viewed in the original work but covers the following major structures:

- Long head of the biceps
- Pectoralis major insertion
- Rotator interval (which includes the supraspinatus, subscapularis, and biceps tendon)
- Coraco-humeral ligament and superior gleno-humeral ligament
- Subscapularis tendon
- Supraspinatus
- Subdeltoid bursa
- Infraspinatus
- Posterior labrum
- Greater tuberosity

A study on the US evaluation of biceps tendon pathology in 71 patients who subsequently underwent arthroscopy found that full-thickness tears and subluxations were identified 100% of the time; however, none of the partial-thickness or intra-articular tears were identified.[2]

US is known to be as accurate as plain radiography for detecting calcium deposits in the rotator cuff without exposing the patient to radiation.[15] Calcific tendinopathy was compared in symptomatic and asymptomatic shoulders using US by Le Goff and colleagues in 2010.[57] They found that subdeltoid-subacromial bursa thickening and power Doppler signal within the calcification were strongly associated with symptomatic calcifications and not associated with asymptomatic calcifications.

Full-thickness rotator cuff tear has a defect from the joint to bursal side of the tendon. Partial tears may show thinning of the bursal surface or focal anechoic or hypoechoic defects.[5] Frequently, secondary signs of rotator cuff tears are often helpful. Full-thickness tears have fluid in the biceps tendon sheath 70% of the time and subdeltoid bursa fluid 85% of the time. Dynamic stressing of the tendon will open a gap in the tendon with full-thickness tears, but not partial tears.[56]

MRI is considered a very accurate method of diagnosing rotator cuff tears, but it is expensive and sometimes contraindicated.[58] Fotiadou and colleagues[17] compared US and MRI with surgical findings in 88 patients. For full-thickness tears, accuracy was 98% for US and 100% for MRI, whereas partial-thickness tears were 87% and 90% respectively. Sipola and colleagues[25] attempted to compare diagnostic US with magnetic resonance angiography (MRA) for detection of rotator cuff tears in 77 patients who had surgical confirmation. They found US sensitivity of 0.92 and specificity of 0.45, compared with MRA sensitivity of 0.97 and specificity of 0.82. Critical appraisal comparing diagnostic US and MRI for rotator cuff tears suggests that additional randomized-controlled studies with larger cohorts are needed for high-level recommendations.[18] A meta-analysis of diagnostic US for subacromial pathology combined data from 23 studies.[59] Full-thickness and partial-thickness tears had enough pooled data to assess the sensitivity and specificity, but other disorders were lacking in enough data to get better assessments. A second meta-analysis that included both published and unpublished data included 62 studies. **Table 2** shows the sensitivity and specificity of several shoulder pathologies from both studies.

Elbow Non-SCI

Musculoskeletal US of the elbow has been shown to be useful to evaluate medial and lateral epicondyles, distal triceps and distal biceps tendons, and effusions.[4] US evaluation of the elbow is done by direct application of the transducer to the tendon, ligament, or joint of interest. Synovial fluid is hypoechoic or anechoic and compressible without Doppler flow.[60] Normal tendon is echogenic longitudinally oriented with fibrillar pattern. Tendon sheaths are hypoechoic lines adjacent to tendon.[19] Tenosynovitis is hypoechoic or anechoic tissue with or without fluid within the tendon sheath that may exhibit Doppler flow pattern.[60]

Table 2
The sensitivities and specificities of diagnostic US for common shoulder pathologies

Pathology	Sensitivity	Specificity
Rotator cuff full-thickness tear	0.95[59] 0.96[26]	0.96[59] 0.93[26]
Rotator cuff partial-thickness tear	0.72[59] 0.84[26]	0.93[59] 0.89[26]
Subacromial bursitis	0.79–0.81[59]	0.94–0.98[59]
Rotator cuff tendinopathy	0.67–0.93[59]	0.88–1.00[59]
Calcific tendinopathy	1.00[59]	0.85–0.98[59]

Several studies have evaluated the sensitivity and specificity of US in lateral epicondylitis. Clarke and colleagues[11] found that larger tears (mean size 8 mm) and lateral collateral ligament tears were associated with poor outcomes with conservative treatments, whereas smaller tears (mean 4 mm) were more likely to improve without surgery. **Table 3** summarizes these findings.

Other pathologies of the elbow have been evaluated by using US as well. Medial epicondylosis has a similar US appearance to lateral epicondylosis.[16] Park and colleagues[61] found US to be 95.2% sensitive, 92% specific, and 93.5% accurate in identifying medial epicondylosis. Although infrequent, a distal triceps tendon full-thickness tear demonstrates a tendon gap; however, partial-thickness tears demonstrate superficial tendon retraction and olecranon enthesophyte avulsion.[14]

Distal biceps tendon tears present with gapping of the tendon, absent tendon, or mass in the antecubital fossa.[6] Partial tears may be difficult to visualize and rely more on indirect measures, such as reduced tendon thickness, hypoechoic appearance, or peritendinous fluid.[20] Lobo Lda and colleagues[62] correlated distal biceps tears identified with US with surgical findings. For the diagnosis of complete versus partial tears, sensitivity was 95% with specificity being 71%; accuracy was 91%. Medial ulnar collateral ligament injury is suited for US, as dynamic valgus stress can widen the ulno-humeral joint compared with the contralateral side.[63] Full-thickness tears are uncommon, although nonvisualization, fluid-filled defects, or avulsed fragments could be seen.[64]

Wrist/Hand Non-SCI

Besides using US to evaluate the median nerve, US of the wrist and hand is used to evaluate tendon ruptures, tendinopathy, pulley injuries, cystic structures, occult fractures, and foreign body localization.[3] Screening of the hand and wrist starts with the hands resting on the examination table. The transducer probe can be placed directly over the tissues to be evaluated. Fingers may be placed in a neutral, slightly flexed position. Contralateral examination allows for comparison.[28] DeQuervain tenosynovitis has hypoechoic thickening of the first extensor compartment with possible effusion or hypervascularity.[29] Studies have shown that US is useful to identify an intracompartmental septum, between the abductor pollicis longus and extensor pollicis brevis tendons, that is frequently seen in DeQuervain tenosynovitis. Choi and colleagues[10] found subcompartmentalization of the first extensor compartment in 73% of surgical DeQuervain tenosynovitis and identified 100% of those who had septums. The same group correctly identified presence or absence of intracompartmental septum in 42 of 43 wrists unresponsive to conservative treatment that had surgery.[65]

Chronic wrist pain is often linked to ganglion cysts. Teefey and colleagues[66] reviewed 84 US examinations on patients with surgery. US correctly identified 87% of cystic lesions, 73% of solid lesions, and 75% of tenosynovitis cases. Chen and colleagues[9] found that 58% of patients with chronic wrist pain had occult ganglion cysts

Table 3
Summary of sensitivities and specificities using US to evaluate lateral epicondylitis

Investigators	Sensitivity	Specificity	Assessment Method
Obradov & Anderson,[22] 2012	0.92–1.00	0.90	Color Doppler and gray-scale combined
	0.50	1.00	Gray-scale calcifications, epicondyle erosions, or hypoechogenic tendons
Lee et al,[21] 2011	0.782	0.952	Common extensor tendon thickness >4.2 mm
	0.863	0.825	Cross-sectional area >32 mm^2

found with US. The use of US to visualize the triangular fibrocartilaginous complex injuries is reported as 63.0% to 87.5% sensitivity with 100% specificity.[23] Few studies comparing US with MRI and arthrogram found US superior in reliability.[23]

Visualization of both extrinsic and intrinsic ligaments of the carpal bones is possible with US with at least partial visibility in nearly all of the major ligaments.[7] However, the radioscapholunate ligament could not be identified; making MRI more useful for some injuries. High-frequency US for identification of early suspected scaphoid fracture was found to have a sensitivity of 78% and a specificity of 89%.[24]

US ELASTOGRAPHY

One of the newer forms of US is elastography US (EUS). Although the technique has been around for in vitro studies since the 1990s,[67–69] it has evolved into an in vivo assessment tool for anatomic structures. Essentially, EUS is a US-based method to quantitatively and qualitatively assess the mechanical properties of different tissues.[67,70,71] There are basically 4 different types of EUS[67]:

- Strain EUS
- Acoustic radiation force impulse (ARFI)
  - A variation of strain EUS
- Shear-wave EUS
- Transient EUS

Strain EUS involves applying a force to the tissue and calculating the axial displacement (strain) before and after compression.[68] This information can be considered qualitative or semiquantitative. In ARFI, the tissue is excited internally with a US pulse. This can access deeper tissues, which may be hard to assess by mechanical compression as in regular-strain EUS.[72] Shear-wave EUS uses the waves generated in tissue by the US pulse from the transducer and has the advantage of being a more objective measure, as it is not dependent on the operator's compression of the tissue.[72,73] Transient EUS is a variation of shear-wave EUS and is also known as vibration-controlled EUS.[74]

These techniques have been used to compare several tendinous structures. In these studies, the symptomatic tendons were found to contain marked softening when compared with asymptomatic tendons.[13,75–77] One study reported the opposite findings with the asymptomatic tendons being softer.[67,78] Besides tendons, the muscle also has the potential to benefit from EUS assessment. There is some evidence that EUS can be used in detecting muscle elasticity changes and help assess for early onset of spasticity.[79]

Given the number of different EUS protocols, and that this is a relatively new technology, there are still some issues with reproducibility, until normal measures can be established. The technical issues include different machines and software,[67] adjacent structures,[80] artifacts, and operator reliability with the amount of compression for strain EUS.[67] Standardization will be needed before this modality can gain widespread use in the SCI population. Because EUS can assess tendons, nerves, and muscles, it has great potential in this population.

SUMMARY

UE pain is common in patients with SCI and can cause significant morbidity. Most structures involved are tendons, ligaments, and nerves. US is a cheap, accurate, and accessible modality to complement the physical examination in these patients. Although current studies have focused on characterizing the changes in patients with SCI with exercise, or comparison of changes with able-bodied control groups, US has the potential to do so much more. There is significant evidence that this modality can recognize the major pathologic processes in the SCI population, but most studies have not included this population. In addition, newer US modalities might be more sensitive in identifying early changes in tendons and nerves, and may lead to early intervention, thus preventing significant morbidity.

REFERENCES

1. Altinok MT, Baysal O, Karakas HM, et al. Sonographic evaluation of the carpal tunnel after provocative exercises. J Ultrasound Med 2004;23:1301–6.
2. Armstrong A, Teefey SA, Wu T, et al. The efficacy of ultrasound in the diagnosis of long head of the biceps tendon pathology. J Shoulder Elbow Surg 2006;15: 7–11.
3. Bajaj S, Pattamapaspong N, Middleton W, et al. Ultrasound of the hand and wrist. J Hand Surg 2009;34:759–60.
4. Beggs I. Ultrasound of the shoulder and elbow. Orthop Clin North Am 2006;37: 277–85, v.
5. Beggs I. Shoulder ultrasound. Seminars Ultrasound Ct MR 2011;32:101–13.
6. Belli P, Costantini M, Mirk P, et al. Sonographic diagnosis of distal biceps tendon rupture: a prospective study of 25 cases. J Ultrasound Med 2001;20:587–95.
7. Boutry N, Lapegue F, Masi L, et al. Ultrasonographic evaluation of normal extrinsic and intrinsic carpal ligaments: preliminary experience. Skeletal Radiol 2005;34:513–21.
8. Brushoj C, Henriksen BM, Albrecht-Beste E, et al. Reproducibility of ultrasound and magnetic resonance imaging measurements of tendon size. Acta Radiol 2006;47:954–9.
9. Chen HS, Chen MY, Lee CY, et al. Ultrasonographic examination on patients with chronic wrist pain: a retrospective study. Am J Phys Med Rehabil 2007;86:907–11.
10. Choi SJ, Ahn JH, Lee YJ, et al. de Quervain disease: US identification of anatomic variations in the first extensor compartment with an emphasis on sub-compartmentalization. Radiology 2011;260:480–6.
11. Clarke AW, Ahmad M, Curtis M, et al. Lateral elbow tendinopathy: correlation of ultrasound findings with pain and functional disability. Am J Sports Med 2010; 38:1209–14.
12. Collinger JL, Gagnon D, Jacobson J, et al. Reliability of quantitative ultrasound mea-sures of the biceps and supraspinatus tendons. Acad Radiol 2009;16:1424–32.
13. De Zordo T, Chhem R, Smekal V, et al. Real-time sonoelastography: findings in patients with symptomatic Achilles tendons and comparison to healthy volun-teers. Ultraschall Med 2010;31:394–400.
14. Downey R, Jacobson JA, Fessell DP, et al. Sonography of partial-thickness tears of the distal triceps brachii tendon. J Ultrasound Med 2011;30:1351–6.
15. Farin PU, Jaroma H. Sonographic findings of rotator cuff calcifications. J Ultrasound Med 1995;14:7–14.
16. Ferrara MA, Marcelis S. Ultrasound of the elbow. J Belge Radiol 1997;80:122–3.
17. Fotiadou AN, Vlychou M, Papadopoulos P, et al. Ultrasonography of symptom-atic rotator cuff tears compared with MR imaging and surgery. Eur J Radiol 2008;68:174–9.
18. Kelly AM, Fessell D. Ultrasound compared with magnetic resonance imaging for the diagnosis of rotator cuff tears: a critically appraised topic. Semin Roentgenol 2009;44:196–200.

19. Lee JC, Healy JC. Normal sonographic anatomy of the wrist and hand. Radiographics 2005;25:1577–90.
20. Lee KS, Rosas HG, Craig JG. Musculoskeletal ultrasound: elbow imaging and procedures. Semin Musculoskelet Radiol 2010;14:449–60.
21. Lee MH, Cha JG, Jin W, et al. Utility of sonographic measurement of the common tensor tendon in patients with lateral epicondylitis. AJR Am J Roentgenol 2011;196:1363–7.
22. Obradov M, Anderson PG. Ultra sonographic findings for chronic lateral epicondylitis. JBR-BTR 2012;95:66–70.
23. Renoux J, Zeitoun-Eiss D, Brasseur JL. Ultrasonographic study of wrist ligaments: review and new perspectives. Semin Musculoskelet Radiol 2009;13:55–65.
24. Senall JA, Failla JM, Bouffard JA, et al. Ultrasound for the early diagnosis of clinically suspected scaphoid fracture. J Hand Surg 2004;29:400–5.
25. Sipola P, Niemitukia L, Kroger H, et al. Detection and quantification of rotator cuff tears with ultrasonography and magnetic resonance imaging—a prospective study in 77 consecutive patients with a surgical reference. Ultrasound Med Biol 2010;36:1981–9.
26. Smith TO, Back T, Toms AP, et al. Diagnostic accuracy of ultrasound for rotator cuff tears in adults: a systematic review and meta-analysis. Clin Radiol 2011;66:1036–48.
27. van Drongelen S, Boninger ML, Impink BG, et al. Ultrasound imaging of acute biceps tendon changes after wheelchair sports. Arch Phys Med Rehabil 2007;88:381–5.
28. Vlad V, Micu M, Porta F, et al. Ultrasound of the hand and wrist in rheumatology. Med Ultrason 2012;14:42–8.
29. Volpe A, Pavoni M, Marchetta A, et al. Ultrasound differentiation of two types of de Quervain's disease: the role of retinaculum. Ann Rheum Dis 2010;69:938–9.
30. Irwin R, Restrepo JA, Sherman A. Musculoskeletal pain in persons with spinal cord injury. Top Spinal Cord Inj Rehabil 2007;13:43–57.
31. Mercer JL, Boninger M, Koontz A, et al. Shoulder joint kinetics and pathology in manual wheelchair users. Clin Biomech (Bristol Avon) 2006;21:781–9.
32. Turner JA, Cardenas DD, Warms CA, et al. Chronic pain associated with spinal cord injuries: a community survey. Arch Phys Med Rehabil 2001;82:501–9.
33. Dalyan M, Cardenas DD, Gerard B. Upper extremity pain after spinal cord injury. Spinal Cord 1999;37:191–5.
34. Dyson-Hudson TA, Kirshblum SC. Shoulder pain in chronic spinal cord injury, part I: epidemiology, etiology, and pathomechanics. J Spinal Cord Med 2004;27:4–17.
35. Subbarao JV, Klopfstein J, Turpin R. Prevalence and impact of wrist and shoulder pain in patients with spinal cord injury. J Spinal Cord Med 1995;18:9–13.
36. Alm M, Saraste H, Norrbrink C. Shoulder pain in persons with thoracic spinal cord injury: prevalence and characteristics. J Rehabil Med 2008;40:277–83.
37. Goldstein B. Musculoskeletal conditions after spinal cord injury. Phys Med Rehabil Clin N Am 2000;11:91–108, viii–ix.
38. Sie IH, Waters RL, Adkins RH, et al. Upper extremity pain in the postrehabilitation spinal cord injured patient. Arch Phys Med Rehabil 1992;73:44–8.
39. Pentland WE, Twomey LT. Upper limb function in persons with long term paraplegia and implications for independence: part I. Paraplegia 1994;32:211–8.
40. Impink BG, Boninger ML, Walker H, et al. Ultrasonographic median nerve changes after a wheelchair sporting event. Arch Phys Med Rehabil 2009;90:1489–94.

41. Dozono K, Hachisuka K, Hatada K, et al. Peripheral neuropathies in the upper extremities of paraplegic wheelchair marathon racers. Paraplegia 1995;33: 208–11.

42. Liang HW, Wang YH, Pan SL, et al. Asymptomatic median mononeuropathy among men with chronic paraplegia. Arch Phys Med Rehabil 2007;88:1193–7.

43. Aljure J, Eltorai I, Bradley WE, et al. Carpal tunnel syndrome in paraplegic patients. Paraplegia 1985;23:182–6.

44. Burnham RS, Steadward RD. Upper extremity peripheral nerve entrapments among wheelchair athletes: prevalence, location, and risk factors. Arch Phys Med Rehabil 1994;75:519–24.

45. Davidoff G, Werner R, Waring W. Compressive mononeuropathies of the upper extremity in chronic paraplegia. Paraplegia 1991;29:17–24.

46. Gellman H, Chandler DR, Petrasek J, et al. Carpal tunnel syndrome in paraplegic patients. J Bone Joint Surg Am 1988;70:517–9.

47. Tun CG, Upton J. The paraplegic hand: electrodiagnostic studies and clinical findings. J Hand Surg 1988;13:716–9.

48. Massy-Westropp N, Grimmer K, Bain G. The effect of a standard activity on the size of the median nerve as determined by ultrasound visualization. J Hand Surg 2001;26:649–54.

49. Maganaris CN, Reeves ND, Rittweger J, et al. Adaptive response of human tendon to paralysis. Muscle Nerve 2006;33:85–92.

50. Dudley-Javoroski S, McMullen T, Borgwardt MR, et al. Reliability and responsiveness of musculoskeletal ultrasound in subjects with and without spinal cord injury. Ultrasound Med Biol 2010;36:1594–607.

51. Kivimaki J, Ahoniemi E. Ultrasonographic findings in shoulders of able-bodied, paraplegic and tetraplegic subjects. Spinal Cord 2008;46:50–2.

52. Brose SW, Boninger ML, Fullerton B, et al. Shoulder ultrasound abnormalities, physical examination findings, and pain in manual wheelchair users with spinal cord injury. Arch Phys Med Rehabil 2008;89:2086–93.

53. Klauser AS, Tagliafico A, Allen GM, et al. Clinical indications for musculoskeletal ultrasound: a Delphi-based consensus paper of the European Society of Musculoskeletal Radiology. Eur Radiol 2012;22:1140–8.

54. Jamadar DA, Jacobson JA, Caoili EM, et al. Musculoskeletal sonography technique: focused versus comprehensive evaluation. AJR Am J Roentgenol 2008; 190:5–9.

55. Nazarian LN, Jacobson JA, Benson CB, et al. Imaging algorithms for evaluating suspected rotator cuff disease: Society of Radiologists in Ultrasound consensus conference statement. Radiology 2013;267:589–95.

56. Allen GM. Shoulder ultrasound imaging—integrating anatomy, biomechanics and disease processes. Eur J Radiol 2008;68:137–46.

57. Le Goff B, Berthelot JM, Guillot P, et al. Assessment of calcific tendonitis of rotator cuff by ultrasonography: comparison between symptomatic and asymptomatic shoulders. Joint Bone Spine 2010;77:258–63.

58. de Jesus JO, Parker L, Frangos AJ, et al. Accuracy of MRI, MR arthrography, and ultrasound in the diagnosis of rotator cuff tears: a meta-analysis. AJR Am J Roentgenol 2009;192:1701–7.

59. Ottenheijm RP, Jansen MJ, Staal JB, et al. Accuracy of diagnostic ultrasound in patients with suspected subacromial disorders: a systematic review and meta-analysis. Arch Phys Med Rehabil 2010;91:1616–25.

60. Wakefield RJ, Balint PV, Szkudlarek M, et al. Musculoskeletal ultrasound including definitions for ultrasonographic pathology. J Rheumatol 2005;32:2485–7.

61. Park GY, Lee SM, Lee MY. Diagnostic value of ultrasonography for clinical medial epicondylitis. Arch Phys Med Rehabil 2008;89:738–42.
62. Lobo Lda G, Fessell DP, Miller BS, et al. The role of sonography in differentiating full versus partial distal biceps tendon tears: correlation with surgical findings. AJR Am J Roentgenol 2013;200:158–62.
63. De Smet AA, Winter TC, Best TM, et al. Dynamic sonography with valgus stress to assess elbow ulnar collateral ligament injury in baseball pitchers. Skeletal Radiol 2002;31:671–6.
64. Miller TT, Adler RS, Friedman L. Sonography of injury of the ulnar collateral ligament of the elbow-initial experience. Skeletal Radiol 2004;33:386–91.
65. Kwon BC, Choi SJ, Koh SH, et al. Sonographic identification of the intracompartmental septum in de Quervain's disease. Clin Orthop Relat Res 2010;468: 2129–34.
66. Teefey SA, Middleton WD, Patel V, et al. The accuracy of high-resolution ultrasound for evaluating focal lesions of the hand and wrist. J Hand Surg 2004; 29:393–9.
67. Drakonaki EE, Allen GM, Wilson DJ. Ultrasound elastography for musculoskeletal applications. Br J Radiol 2012;85:1435–45.
68. Ophir J, Cespedes I, Ponnekanti H, et al. Elastography: a quantitative method for imaging the elasticity of biological tissues. Ultrason Imaging 1991;13: 111–34.
69. Lerner RM, Huang SR, Parker KJ. "Sonoelasticity" images derived from ultrasound signals in mechanically vibrated tissues. Ultrasound Med Biol 1990;16: 231–9.
70. Garra BS. Imaging and estimation of tissue elasticity by ultrasound. Ultrasound Q 2007;23:255–68.
71. Garra BS. Elastography: current status, future prospects, and making it work for you. Ultrasound Q 2011;27:177–86.
72. Li Y, Snedeker JG. Elastography: modality-specific approaches, clinical applications, and research horizons. Skeletal Radiol 2011;40:389–97.
73. Bercoff J, Tanter M, Fink M. Supersonic shear imaging: a new technique for soft tissue elasticity mapping. IEEE Trans Ultrason Ferroelectr Freq Control 2004;51: 396–409.
74. Sandrin L, Fourquet B, Hasquenoph JM, et al. Transient elastography: a new noninvasive method for assessment of hepatic fibrosis. Ultrasound Med Biol 2003;29:1705–13.
75. De Zordo T, Fink C, Feuchtner GM, et al. Real-time sonoelastography findings in healthy Achilles tendons. AJR Am J Roentgenol 2009;193:W134–8.
76. Klauser AS, Faschingbauer R, Jaschke WR. Is sonoelastography of value in assessing tendons? Semin Musculoskelet Radiol 2010;14:323–33.
77. De Zordo T, Lill SR, Fink C, et al. Real-time sonoelastography of lateral epicondylitis: comparison of findings between patients and healthy volunteers. AJR Am J Roentgenol 2009;193:180–5.
78. Sconfienza LM, Silvestri E, Cimmino MA. Sonoelastography in the evaluation of painful Achilles tendon in amateur athletes. Clin Exp Rheumatol 2010;28:373–8.
79. Vasilescu D, Vasilescu D, Dudea S, et al. Sonoelastography contribution in cerebral palsy spasticity treatment assessment, preliminary report: a systematic review of the literature apropos of seven patients. Med Ultrason 2010;12:306–10.
80. Bhatia KS, Rasalkar DD, Lee YP, et al. Real-time qualitative ultrasound elastography of miscellaneous non-nodal neck masses: applications and limitations. Ultrasound Med Biol 2010;36:1644–52.

Chronic Neuropathic Pain in SCI: Evaluation and Treatment

 CrossMark

Elizabeth Roy Felix, PhD[a,b],*

KEYWORDS

- Neuropathic pain • Pain management • Pharmacologic treatment
- Nonpharmacologic treatment • Pain evaluation

KEY POINTS

- Chronic neuropathic pain after a spinal cord injury (SCI) is common and difficult to treat in many patients. The evaluation and proper diagnosis of the pain conditions of patients with SCI are especially important in this patient group in order to make informed treatment decisions.
- The use of validated assessment tools and questionnaires in clinical practice can help the physiatrist track outcomes when new treatment approaches are embarked on and offer an avenue for enriched discussion with, and evaluation of, patients in pain.
- Although studies of the long-term efficacy of pharmacologic agents for pain management in patients with SCI and neuropathic pain are lacking, strong support for the safety and efficacy of pregabalin does exist. Gabapentin, amitriptyline, and duloxetine have less support but may be effective in some patients.
- Even fewer clinical trials exist for nonpharmacologic treatment strategies, such as massage, acupuncture, and transcutaneous, spinal, and transcranial stimulation, although survey studies show that persons with SCI and chronic pain are receptive to such therapies and often report good outcomes.

INTRODUCTION

The presence of chronic pain in patients with spinal cord injury (SCI) is the rule, not the exception, with most studies estimating that approximately 70% of individuals with SCI have persistent pain[1–5] that does not subside with time.[6,7] The impact that chronic pain has on emotional function, activities of daily living, and quality of life in those patients with SCI is well documented.[8]

Chronic pain after SCI is most commonly either nociceptive or neuropathic in nature. The mechanisms and treatment approaches for nociceptive pains are typically

Disclosure: The author has no financial disclosures.
[a] Department of Physical Medicine & Rehabilitation, University of Miami Miller School of Medicine, PO Box 016960, C-206, Miami, FL 33101, USA; [b] Research Service, Department of Veterans Affairs Medical Center, Miami VAHS, 1201 North West 16th Street, Miami, FL 33125, USA
* Department of Physical Medicine & Rehabilitation, University of Miami Miller School of Medicine, PO Box 016960, C-206, Miami, FL 33101.
E-mail address: efelix@med.miami.edu

more easily identified than those for neuropathic pains; although the prevalence of chronic neuropathic pain in persons with SCI is lower (approximately 40%[6,9,10]) than for nociceptive pains, it is generally rated as more severe.[6]

The possible symptoms and signs for neuropathic pain are shown in **Box 1**. An individual with neuropathic pain may exhibit all or only a few of these components of neuropathic pain. Typically, a patient will complain of spontaneous burning pain that is continuously present and may be accompanied by dysesthesias often described as tingling or pricking. He or she may also describe electric shock–like or stabbing sensations that are intermittent and may or may not be provoked by stimulation. Some patients will also describe being especially sensitive in the area of neuropathic pain, referring to pain that is induced by light touch or moderate thermal stimuli (ie, allodynia) and to particularly severe pain elicited by normally mild nociceptive stimuli (ie, hyperalgesia).

Much research has been devoted to understanding the mechanisms of neuropathic pain and investigating the efficacy of several treatment options so that most patients who develop this type of pain might realize the reduction or elimination of pain. Although neuropathic pain caused by SCI shares some mechanisms with neuropathic pain of other origins, several treatments that have been shown to be effective in other patient groups, particularly those with peripheral neuropathic pain, have been less effective for individuals with SCI.

Suggestions for the proper evaluation of patients with SCI who have pain; for treatment approaches, both pharmacologic and nonpharmacologic; and for monitoring the efficacy of treatments in patients with pain are presented in this review. Definitions for the pain terminology used can be found in **Box 2**.

PATIENT EVALUATION OVERVIEW
Comprehensive Evaluation of Patients in Pain

It has often been suggested that patients with chronic pain need to be evaluated and treated with several factors in mind, including the potential cause of pain; the severity of pain; the functional limitations caused by pain; and the history, psychology, behavior, and cultural characteristics of the patients. Considering the complexity of

---

Box 1
Typical symptoms and signs of neuropathic pain

Spontaneous pain

- Burning, pricking
- Nonpainful sensations (tingling, itching)
- Continuous
- Intermittent/paroxysmal

Evoked pain

- Allodynia
- Hyperalgesia
- Tactile
- Thermal

Neuropathic pain is generally identified by its spontaneous pain characteristics, which may include all or some of the qualities listed. Exaggerated pain provoked by tactile or thermal stimuli is present in many, but not all, cases of neuropathic pain.

Box 2
Pain definitions

Pain: An unpleasant sensory and emotional experience associated with actual or potential tissue damage or described in terms of such damage[134]

Nociceptive pain: Pain that arises from actual or threatened damage to non-neural tissue and is caused by the activation of nociceptors[134]

Neuropathic pain: Pain arising as a direct consequence of a lesion or disease affecting the somatosensory system[14]

Spontaneous pain: Pain that is not evoked by a known stimulus

Evoked pain: Pain that is caused by an external stimulus

Allodynia: Pain caused by a stimulus that does not normally provoke pain[134]

Hyperalgesia: Increased pain from a stimulus that normally provokes pain[134]

Dysesthesia: An unpleasant abnormal sensation, whether spontaneous or evoked (can include allodynia or hyperalgesia)[134]

---

health, social, and psychological issues that patients with SCI face, this global approach is especially important.[11] In order to best select and evaluate treatments, therefore, the clinician should include several assessments, targeting different domains of the pain experience, and not concentrate only on the reduction of pain intensity when determining treatment efficacy in patients.[12–14]

Establishing a Diagnosis of Neuropathic Pain in SCI

Chronic pain conditions can result from several causes; signs and symptoms of the same underlying pathophysiology may differ from patient to patient, thus, establishing that a patient's reported pain is neuropathic in nature is not always straightforward. The criteria for determining a diagnosis of neuropathic pain were proposed by the Special Interest Group on Neuropathic Pain (NeuPSIG) of the International Association for the Study of Pain (IASP) in 2008.[15] This group of experts suggested a grading system of *definite*, *probable*, and *possible* neuropathic pain. According to their published criteria, a *definite* neuropathic pain diagnosis would require (1) a pain distribution consistent with injury to the peripheral nervous system (PNS) or the central nervous system (CNS), (2) a previous or current injury or disease affecting the PNS and/or CNS, (3) abnormal sensory signs within the body area corresponding to the injured part of the CNS or PNS, and (4) a diagnostic test confirming a lesion or disease in these structures. Based on these definitions, almost any pain reported at and/or below the neurologic level of injury in a person with SCI would qualify as a neuropathic pain. This general definition of neuropathic pain could be especially problematic for pains located at the level of injury, in which sensory dysfunction (requirement [3] of the aforementioned definition) could be present in an area where either or both nociceptive and neuropathic mechanisms underlie the pain report.[16,17] Taking this into account, Finnerup and Baastrup[18] added additional criteria for neuropathic pain specifically for persons with SCI: (1) onset of pain within 1 year following SCI; (2) no primary relation to movement, inflammation, or other local tissue damage; and (3) hot-burning, tingling, pricking, pins-and-needles, sharp, shooting, squeezing, cold, electric, or shock-like quality of pain.

Based on these criteria, a determination of a probable neuropathic pain diagnosis can be made by a careful examination and interview of patients with SCI, which can be assisted by using validated self-report measures, some of which are specifically targeted toward neuropathic pain characteristics (**Table 1**; also see "Tools for Diagnosis and

Table 1
Select tools for a comprehensive evaluation of neuropathic pain in patients with SCI

Type of Assessment	Measurement Tool	Description
Neuropathic pain screening These assessments can be used as initial screening tools for the possible presence of neuropathic pain in patients with SCI.	Neuropathic Pain Questionnaire[135]	12 items assessing the presence and severity of different qualities of pain and sensations associated with neuropathic pain; includes 2 affective aspects (unpleasant, overwhelming); sensitivity = 66%, specificity = 75%
	Pain-DETECT[136]	9 items regarding symptoms associated with neuropathic pain; 2 items regarding presence of evoked sensations; ≥19 = neuropathic pain likely; ≤12 = neuropathic pain unlikely; sensitivity = 85%, specificity = 80%
	ID Pain[137]	6 items used to discriminate between neuropathic and nociceptive pain; >3 = likely presence of neuropathic pain
	Leeds Assessment of Neuropathic Symptoms and Signs[29]	7 items: 5 self-report symptoms and 2 physical assessments for brush allodynia and pinprick hyperalgesia; ≥12 = neuropathic pain likely; sensitivity = 85%, specificity = 80%
	Douleur Neuropathique en 4 questions[30]	10-item questionnaire and assessment; 7 self-report items of the presence of specific pain qualities associated with neuropathic pain and 3 physical examination items for decreased sensitivity to touch and pinprick and allodynia to brushing; >4 = likely neuropathic pain; sensitivity = 83%, specificity = 90%
Pain intensity These scales are used in the clinic and in research as primary outcome measures regarding the effectiveness of treatments. Patients are typically asked to rate the intensity of their pain on average.	Numerical rating scale	0–10 scale, where 0 typically means no pain and 10 is typically defined as the most intense pain imaginable; patients must choose a number to represent the intensity of their pain
	Visual analog scale	10-cm horizontal line is presented to patients, with "no pain" as an anchor at the left end and "the most intense pain imaginable" as an anchor on the right end of the line; patients are instructed to estimate pain intensity by marking on the line the place where pain intensity falls
	Verbal rating scale	Patients choose a word/phrase to indicate pain intensity: no pain, slight pain, mild pain, moderate pain, severe pain, extreme pain, the most intense pain imaginable

Characteristics/severity of neuropathic pain These questionnaires are scored to evaluate the severity of symptoms associated with neuropathic pain.	Neuropathic Pain Scale[32]	1 item to rate overall intensity of pain; 6 items to assess the intensity of separate qualities of pain (eg, burning, sharp, itchy); 1 item to assess temporal aspects of pain; 1 item to rate unpleasantness of pain; and separate ratings for the intensity of surface and deep pain
	Neuropathic Pain Symptom Inventory[33]	10 items for rating the intensity of different qualities or evoked aspects of pain; 2 items to evaluate temporal aspects of pain; 5 subscale scores can be calculated as well as a total score
Impact of pain on function These assessment tools are used to evaluate the extent to which pain interferes with activities or other aspects of life.	Interference subscale of the Brief Pain Inventory–short form[34]	7 items to rate regarding the interference of pain on activities, sleep, mood, and relationships; a revised version for patients with disability has been published[138]
	Life Interference subscale of the Multidimensional Pain Inventory[139]	Assesses activities of daily living and social aspects (relationships with family, friends) regarding the impact that pain has on the satisfaction or enjoyment of each activity/relationship; a revised version for use with patients who have SCI has been published[140]
Emotional function Each questionnaire is scored to obtain an estimate of the severity of different emotional and psychological aspects of patients with neuropathic pain.	Beck Depression Inventory[38]	21 items scored on a 0-4 scale, with higher scores indicating greater depressive symptoms; scores ≥ 17 are considered borderline, or worse, clinical depression
	Spielberger State-Trait Anxiety Inventory[39]	20 items are rated to evaluate state anxiety and 20 items are rated to evaluate trait anxiety
	Hospital Anxiety and Depression Scale[40]	7 items evaluate anxiety and 7 items evaluate depression; can be used to evaluate the extent of anxiety and depressive symptoms in patients
	Pain Catastrophizing Scale[41]	13 items each rated on a 5-point scale to evaluate the extent the individual engages in catastrophic thinking with regards to pain; a total score and 3 subscale scores (rumination, magnification, helplessness) can be calculated
Impression of change/evaluation of outcome This tool evaluates a patient's perspective on the improvement or worsening of his/her condition after a treatment approach has been tried	Patient Global Impression of Change	Typically one question is used that is suited to the situation (eg, Compared with the time before you started this medication, how would you rate your condition now?); response categories are provided ranging from very much improved to very much worse

Evaluation of Neuropathic Pain" section later). Additionally, the presentation of select stimuli to evaluate positive or negative sensory signs (ie, hyposensitivities or hypersensitivities) in areas where spontaneous pain is reported will yield further insight.[19]

SCI Pain Taxonomy

It is important to note that most patients with SCI have more than one persistent pain problem,[20–22] so differentiating between a patient's pains, with respect to location, quality, and factors that increase or decrease the pain, is particularly important for comprehensive pain management. This necessity is evident in the International Spinal Cord Injury Basic Pain Dataset (ISCIBPD)[21,23,24] and the International Spinal Cord Injury Pain (ISCIP) Classification,[25,26] which require that each pain that an individual experiences is evaluated separately in order to best define a patient's pain profile.

The ISCIP Classification, published in 2012,[25] is an attempt by international experts in the SCI and pain community to develop a consensus classification scheme so that research and clinical efforts are not confused by differences in nomenclature or criteria. The ISCIP Classification consists of a 3-tiered structure, with the first tier differentiating nociceptive, neuropathic, other, and unknown pain. In accordance with the IASP's definitions, the ISCIP Classification identifies nociceptive pain as pain that is caused by the activation of nociceptors and neuropathic pain as pain that is caused by a lesion or disease of the somatosensory nervous system.[25,27] The ISCIP defines other pain as pain that does not have an identifiable cause attributable to nociceptive or neuropathic mechanisms and is unrelated to SCI onset but that has been defined (eg, fibromyalgia, complex regional pain syndrome type I). Unknown pain types are those pains for which nociceptive, neuropathic, or other cannot be reasonably assigned.

It is recognized in the ISCIP Classification that a pain located in the same or overlapping areas can be classified as having more than one component (eg, nociceptive and neuropathic) based on the presenting signs and symptoms as well as imaging diagnostics. The primary reason for identifying different types of pains using a consensus classification scheme is so that the principal mechanisms causing the pain may be identified and studied and, thus, treatment approaches can be better selected and evaluated.

Types of Neuropathic Pain in Patients with SCI

In addition to establishing a probable diagnosis of neuropathic pain, it is further helpful to determine whether the pain is located in the region above, at, and/or below the level of injury and whether it is likely to be peripheral or central in nature. Identifying these features of pain can aid in choosing viable treatment options.

Tier 2 of the ISCIP Classification further divides the tier 1 classifications of nociceptive pain and neuropathic pain. The tier 2 subcategories for neuropathic pain are at-level SCI pain, below-level SCI pain, and other neuropathic pain (not directly related to the SCI). The descriptions for and examples of each of these subcategories can be found in **Table 2**. The identification of the source of the pain and/or the underlying pathologic condition(s) is recommended as the tier 3 level of classification, if possible.[25] The tier 3 classification would necessarily be influenced by imaging and additional diagnostic tests and would further guide the clinician in selecting management strategies.

Tools for Diagnosis and Evaluation of Neuropathic Pain

As mentioned previously, it is particularly important in persons with SCI to determine whether more than one pain is present and to ask patients to identify characteristics of each pain separately. Based on the published guidelines for the evaluation of pain both

Table 2
Neuropathic pain subtypes in SCI according to the ISCIP classification

Tier 2 Subcategory of Neuropathic Pain in SCI	Description/Criteria	Example Pathologic Condition(s) or Source of Pain/Tier 3
At-level SCI pain	• Lesion or disease of the nerve root (peripheral nervous system) or spinal cord (central nervous system) resulting in segmental pattern of pain • Location of pain within the dermatome of the NLI and the 3 levels below the NLI but not present in lower dermatomes (exception: if cauda equine damage is presumed cause, then pain can include areas more than 3 levels below the NLI) • Sensory deficits likely within the reported pain area • Allodynia and/or hyperalgesia may be present within reported pain area • Pain described as hot-burning, tingling, pricking, pins and needles, sharp, shooting, squeezing painful cold, and electric shock–like	• Spinal cord compression • Nerve root injury • Cauda equina injury
Below-level SCI pain	• Pain caused by SCI (central nervous system); pain distribution includes areas more than 3 dermatomes below the NLI • May also include areas at the NLI and within the 3 dermatomes below the NLI • Sensory deficits likely within the reported pain area • Allodynia and/or hyperalgesia may be present within the reported pain area • Pain described as hot-burning, tingling, pricking, pins and needles, sharp, shooting, squeezing painful cold, and electric shock–like	• Spinal cord lesion
Other neuropathic pain	• Pain not thought to be associated with the SCI • Pain distribution can be located above, at, or below the NLI • Sensory deficits as well as allodynia and hyperalgesia may be present in the reported painful area • Pain described as hot-burning, tingling, pricking, pins and needles, sharp, shooting, squeezing painful cold, and electric shock–like	• Carpel tunnel compression • Diabetic neuropathy

Abbreviation: NLI, neurologic level of injury.
Data from Bryce TN, Biering-Sørensen F, Finnerup NB, et al. International SCI pain classification: part I. Background and description. Spinal Cord 2012;50:413–7.

in patient groups with mixed causes of neuropathic pain[14] and specifically in patients with SCI-related neuropathic pain,[13] the global evaluation of pain characteristics should include pain intensity, temporal aspects of pain, pain qualities, impact of pain on activities of daily living and quality of life, and the psychological state of the person in pain.

The ISCIPBD tool[24] may be useful to provide the clinical team with a standardized pain evaluation form to start with. This form includes the patient's report regarding the impact of pain on sleep, mood, and activities; identification of areas of the body where pain is present; pain intensity ratings; classification of pain; onset of pain; and whether or not medications are currently used for pain.

Several recommended measures for assessing overall functioning in patients with pain are outlined later and included in **Table 1**. A battery of these questionnaires should be considered by the clinical team regardless of whether a patient is partici-pating in a clinical trial, as these validated questionnaires can help to better under-stand the impact that pain has on the life of the patient and provide standardized baseline assessments that may be used for comparison during follow-up visits, partic-ularly when a new treatment approach is being embarked on.

Screening tools for diagnosing neuropathic pain

Several screening tools have been developed by different groups as a way to initially identify patients that may have neuropathic pain. They are listed and described in **Table 1**. The use of these tools provides an easy way to initially identify patients that may have neuropathic pain, but they fail to identify about 10% to 20% of persons who would be diagnosed with neuropathic pain based on a pain specialist's diag-nosis.[14] These screening tools all ask patients to describe their pain in terms of qual-ities that have long been associated with neuropathic pain[28] and 2 (Leeds Assessment of Neuropathic Symptoms and Signs,[29] Douleur Neuropathique en 4 questions [DN4][30]) also include an assessment component (measurement of evoked sensations) that should be carried out by the examiner. No recommendation was made by the NeuPSIG of the IASP as to which specific neuropathic pain screening tool should be used,[14] but a systematic review regarding neuropathic pain in SCI recommended the DN4, as it has evidenced high sensitivity (89.9%) and specificity (82.9%).[13]

For a diagnosis of neuropathic pain, it is required that the pain be located in an area of sensory disturbance.[15] Therefore, a proper neurologic examination (ie, International Standards for Neurologic Classification of Spinal Cord Injury[31]) is critical to identify whether the pain is in an area affected by the spinal cord lesion; classification at the tier 2 level (at, below, other) in the ISCIP Classification[25,26] terminology also requires the establishment of the level of injury.

Quantitative sensory testing (QST) has recently been endorsed as a complementary tool to the clinical examination for obtaining additional information regarding the func-tional status of the somatosensory system.[19] A few studies have shown that results from QST vary with treatment effects and can be used to predict the treatment outcome.[14] However, universally accepted standards for performing QST in the clin-ical setting do not currently exist, making the use of QST for diagnostic purposes premature.

Tools for capturing the severity and characteristics of neuropathic pain

The most common, and recommended, tool used to evaluate pain intensity for research or clinical purposes is the numerical rating scale (NRS). The visual analog scale (VAS) and the verbal rating scale are also often used. In order to obtain a picture of the severity of a patient's pain, it is recommended that patients are asked to rate the intensity of their pain when it is at its worst, at its least, and on average.[14]

Evaluating the components of neuropathic pain, including the spontaneous, continuous, intermittent, and evoked aspects, may yield additional insights regarding possible treatment choices and the effect of treatments on each component separately, as they may be the result of independent mechanisms that are differentially affected by the treatment. The Neuropathic Pain Scale[32] and the Neuropathic Pain Symptom Inventory (NPSI)[33] (see **Table 1**) were created to assess the severity and temporal aspects of common symptoms of neuropathic pain. The NPSI has been recommended in both the NeuPSIG's guidelines[14] and in the review by Calmels and colleagues,[13] which was specifically geared toward SCI-related neuropathic pain.

Tools to evaluate the impact of pain on physical function
The effect that neuropathic pain has on the ability to perform activities of daily living in persons with SCI should be evaluated separately from the effects that are caused by limitations in motor function. The Brief Pain Inventory (short form)[34] interference subscale is frequently used for this purpose, although it includes one item (interference with walking ability) that is not appropriate for most patients with SCI. It has been endorsed by several groups[13,14,35] and can be used to track the extent of disability caused by neuropathic pain across different time periods, so that the impact a pain management strategy has on physical function can be assessed.

Tools for evaluating emotional function
The preexisting psychological state of a patient in pain has been shown to be an indicator of the success of particular treatment approaches.[36,37] Thus, it is prudent to evaluate depression, anxiety, and pain coping style in patients with SCI and neuropathic pain. By asking only general questions about the presence of psychological concerns, an examiner may overlook clinically significant symptoms of psychological distress. Therefore, the use of validated screening assessments and questionnaires may assist with treatment decisions and referrals, if necessary.

Recommendations for the assessment of psychological function in patients with chronic pain[13,14,35] include the following: Beck Depression Inventory,[38] Spielberger State-Trait Anxiety Inventory,[39] Hospital Anxiety and Depression Scale,[40] and the Pain Catastrophizing Scale (see **Table 1**).[41]

It may not be practical to use all of the assessments and questionnaires identified here in the clinical setting. However, the administration of a selection of these measures to patients on the initial evaluation can assist the clinician in his or her decision making regarding the best strategies for pain management. In addition, follow-up using the same questionnaires can provide a concrete and less biased way of evaluating treatment efficacy compared with a general question of how patients are doing.

PHARMACOLOGIC TREATMENT OPTIONS

The treatment of neuropathic pain conditions is notoriously difficult,[42] and neuropathic pain after SCI is especially refractory to treatment.[43–45] Many of the pharmacologic approaches that have been tested for SCI pain were first shown to be effective for peripheral neuropathic pain conditions[46] and, thus, may not target the primary mechanisms responsible for SCI-associated neuropathic pain. Even those pharmacologic treatments that have been shown to provide effective relief or reduction in pain for many individuals with SCI are found by other individuals either to not provide sufficient relief or to produce side effects that are intolerable.[44,45] An overview of the pharmacologic agents that show the most promise for treating neuropathic pain in persons with SCI are listed in **Table 3**. Evidence for the efficacy of these medications, and others, is reviewed in the following text.

Table 3
Select pharmacologic treatments for neuropathic pain in SCI

Medication	Typical Dosage Range (Per Day)	Common Side Effects	Special Considerations
Anticonvulsants			
Gabapentin	400–3600 mg	Somnolence, dizziness, diarrhea, constipation, peripheral edema, asthenia, weight gain, dry mouth	• Should consider renal function when choosing dose
Pregabalin	150–600 mg	Somnolence, dizziness, peripheral edema, asthenia, dry mouth, constipation	• May be contraindicated in patients with heart conditions, renal insufficiency • Effect may be seen as quickly as 1 wk • FDA approved for treatment of SCI neuropathic pain
Antidepressants			
Amitriptyline	125–150 mg	Dry mouth, orthostatic hypotension, constipation	• May be contraindicated in patients with ischemic cardiac disease; screening electrocardiogram is recommended for patients older than 40 y • May be most effective in patients with comorbid depressive symptoms
Venlafaxine	150–250 mg	Nausea, headache, sedation, dizziness	• Should monitor changes in blood pressure during treatment • May be contraindicated in patients with cardiac disease • Should use slow tapering to avoid possible withdrawal syndrome
Duloxetine	60–120 mg	Somnolence, nausea-vomiting, dizziness, confusion, headache	• Use cautiously in patients with seizures or a bleeding tendency • Should monitor blood pressure during treatment
Opioids			
Tramadol	100–400 mg	Somnolence, dry mouth, dizziness, sweating, constipation, nausea	• Side effects may be intolerable • Not suggested as a long-term treatment strategy

Abbreviation: FDA, Food and Drug Administration.

Anticonvulsants

Anticonvulsant, or antiepileptic, medications include a variety of pharmacologic agents. The general mechanism of anticonvulsants is to prevent excessive neuronal firing, which seems to be a common link between epileptic seizure disorders and chronic neuropathic pain; but the specific mechanisms of action differ considerably among the agents within this class of drugs.

Anticonvulsants are used by many patients with neuropathic pain after SCI.[22,44] Gabapentin and pregabalin are generally considered first-line agents for the treatment of SCI-associated neuropathic pain[46,47] and have been the most studied anticonvulsants in patients with SCI.

Pregabalin, whose mechanism of action is similar to that of gabapentin, has been shown to be effective in 2 large (n>100) placebo-controlled multisite clinical trials in patients with SCI and neuropathic pain.[48,49] The average reduction in pain across these studies was 1.92 and 1.66 on a 0 to 10 rating scale, respectively, with a number needed to treat (NNT) (for a 50% pain reduction) of approximately 7 in both studies. A smaller study (n = 40), which included patients with central neuropathic pain of different causes (approximately 50% were subjects with SCI), further supports the efficacy of pregabalin, showing a reduction in pain rating of 2.5 during the 4-week trial.[50] Based on evidence from these studies, pregabalin was recently approved by the Food and Drug Administration specifically for its use in patients with SCI and neuropathic pain, after having been previously approved for neuropathic pain associated with diabetic peripheral neuropathy and postherpetic neuralgia.[51]

Gabapentin has shown efficacy in reducing pain intensity in patients with neuropathic pain after SCI in small clinical trials (n<30),[52,53] with an additional study reporting significant decreases in "unpleasant feelings" in subjects treated with gabapentin compared with subjects randomized to placebo (with trends for reductions in pain intensity and burning feeling).[54] A retrospective chart review[55] and an observational study[56] additionally support the efficacy of gabapentin in patients with SCI. However, Rintala and colleagues[57] found gabapentin to be no more effective than amitriptyline or an active placebo (diphenhydramine) in a blinded crossover trial of 38 subjects.[57]

Other anticonvulsants that may be prescribed for neuropathic pain after SCI generally have little or no support for their efficacy in the literature. Levetiracetam was found to provide no significant improvement in pain intensity compared with placebo in a randomized crossover controlled trial in subjects with SCI and neuropathic pain.[58] Similarly, valproate[59] and lamotrigine[60] did not produce significant effects compared with placebo in randomized controlled trials, although subgroup analyses did show significant pain reduction with lamotrigine in subjects with SCI who had incomplete lesions (n = 12).[60] Additionally, carbamazepine did not confer any protective effect for the development of neuropathic pain in newly injured patients with SCI[61]; this medication has not been tested in a clinical trial in patients with established chronic neuropathic pain after SCI. The potential effectiveness of anticonvulsants when combined with other pharmacologic treatments has some support in the literature (see "Combination therapies"), but these effects have not been confirmed by a double-blind randomized controlled trial in patients with SCI-associated neuropathic pain.

Antidepressants

It has been suggested that the analgesic effects of certain antidepressant drugs on neuropathic pain rely on different mechanisms of action than those that are related to their antidepressant effects. This finding is attributable to the fact that the doses needed for pain relief are generally subclinical for producing antidepressant effects, and analgesic effects can be seen weeks before improvement in depressive symtpoms.[62] Tricyclic antidepressants (TCAs) and serotonin-norepinephrine reuptake inhibitors (SNRIs) are the most common antidepressant agents used by those with SCI-associated chronic pain.

The relative popularity of amitriptyline, a TCA, for the treatment of neuropathic pain after SCI is likely because of its proven effectiveness in patients with other neuropathic pain conditions (eg, diabetic neuropathy, postherpetic neuralgia), though it is suggested that amitriptyline provides sufficient relief in only a minority of these patients (approximately 25%[63]). TCAs have been suggested as first-line agents for neuropathic pain (not specific to SCI) by experts in the field[42,64] and may be effective in select patients with SCI-related neuropathic pain if side effects are tolerable. Two double-blind controlled studies of amitriptyline for pain relief specifically in persons with SCI did not find significant reductions in pain with treatment,[57,65] although a subgroup analysis in one of the studies showed a significant reduction of pain in those subjects who also had depressive symptoms.[57]

SNRIs are relatively recent additions to the neuropathic pain arsenal, and their potential utility as a treatment for neuropathic pain in SCI is largely based on clinical trial results and anecdotal success in other neuropathic pain conditions. Duloxetine has been shown to be an effective analgesic in several controlled trials in diabetic peripheral neuropathy,[42] with an NNT of approximately 5 in this patient population.[66] A recent study of duloxetine in patients with severe chronic central neuropathic pain (71% SCI) showed a trend ($P = .05$) for significantly greater improvement in VAS scores for pain intensity for the group administered 8 weeks of 60 to 120 mg/d compared with the group administered placebo.[67] Additionally, the Patient Global Impression of Change (PGIC) was significantly different between the groups, with those subjects in the duloxetine arm reporting greater improvement of their situation at the end of the study ($P = .014$).[67]

Venlafaxine has shown efficacy for reducing pain in a few controlled trials in patients with pain associated with polyneuropathy, both for patients with diabetes-associated neuropathy[68] and for patients with other causes of neuropathy.[69] Based on the positive results seen for venlafaxine and duloxetine, and their relatively modest side-effect profiles, they have been recommended as first-line treatments for neuropathic pain in general[64]; but clinical trials of venlafaxine in patients with SCI-associated neuropathic pain have not yet been published.

Opioids

Tramadol is the only orally administered opioid that has been tested in a randomized controlled trial in persons with SCI and neuropathic pain. In this study, subjects were persons with chronic SCI (average 14.6 years after injury) who had chronic neuropathic pain at or below the level of injury for at least 6 months.[70] After a 4-week intervention of either tramadol (100–400 mg/d) or placebo, the subjects in the tramadol arm had a significantly greater reduction of pain than those in the placebo arm. However, 43% of subjects who began treatment on tramadol withdrew from the study before the end of the 4-week treatment period because of adverse side effects compared with 17% of the subjects administered placebo. The efficacy of tramadol in other neuropathic pain patient populations has also been supported in placebo-controlled studies.[71] Tramadol may be a viable treatment option for those patients with SCI-associated neuropathic pain that is refractory to first-line treatments and for whom the adverse events are tolerable.[47]

Support for the efficacy of oxycodone as an analgesic in patients with neuropathic pain associated with postherpetic neuralgia or diabetic neuropathy is present in the literature.[42] One prospective, observational study lends moderate support for its use in patients with SCI and neuropathic pain, showing significant decreases in VAS ratings of pain intensity and increases in quality of life over the course of a 3-month follow-up period.[72] Only 2 subjects withdrew based on adverse effects; but 33.3% of subjects complained of constipation, the most frequent side effect.[72] Given the low level of evidence provided by this observational study, it is difficult to determine whether oxycodone will prove effective for the treatment of neuropathic pain associated with SCI.

There is some support for the use of opioids administered intravenously for the relief of pain associated with SCI. An early study in 9 patients with SCI pain found that intravenous (IV) alfentanil (μ-opioid agonist) was effective at significantly reducing ongoing pain, allodynia, and wind-up–like pain. Similarly, Attal and colleagues[73] reported that in their sample of patients with central pain (after stroke or SCI), IV morphine (μ-opioid agonist) produced a significantly greater reduction in evoked pain sensations (allodynia) compared with placebo. However, they did not find a significantly greater reduction in intensity ratings of spontaneous pain for morphine compared with placebo.[73] Additionally, those subjects who did report reductions in ongoing pain with IV morphine were more likely to report pain reduction when given oral morphine compared with nonresponders to IV morphine and to continue taking oral morphine when assessed 1 year later.[73]

The effect of intrathecal (IT) or epidural administration of morphine has been reported in the literature, with a randomized blinded study reporting no effect with a single IT injection in 15 patients with SCI[74]; a study of the pain-relieving effects of lidocaine, morphine, and clonidine in subjects with SCI and refractory pain reported mixed results.[75] Although some subjects obtained substantial pain relief, it was short lived. Given the lack of consistent results across studies, and the short duration of its analgesic effect, injections or infusions of opioids for relief of neuropathic pain after SCI are not recommended as a long-term management strategy.

Cannabinoids

Although survey studies of persons with SCI and chronic pain support the use of cannabinoids for the relief of pain,[22,45] there is scant literature regarding its efficacy in clinical trials. One small study of dronabinol did not show efficacy compared with an active placebo in patients with SCI pain.[76]

The results from small (n<40) clinical trials in other neuropathic pain patient groups, and in studies with mixed diagnoses that include SCI-related neuropathic pain, generally support the use of cannabis or cannabinoid agents for at least modest reductions in pain intensity and improvements in secondary outcomes (eg, sleep, mood),[77–79] although one large study (n = 339) reported equivocal results.[80] The efficacy of different doses of tetrahydrocannabinol (THC) for the reduction of neuropathic pain suggests that low doses can confer similar analgesic effects as medium and high doses, and low-dose THC limits the effect of the drug on cognitive decline.[77,79]

Studies that did report significant effects of cannabinoids on neuropathic pain included both subjects with central neuropathic pain and subjects with peripheral neuropathic pain,[77–79] whereas the large study that did not show definitive effects of THC compared with placebo was limited to those with central neuropathic pain caused by multiple sclerosis. Given the generally tolerable side-effect profile for low-dose THC, future randomized controlled trials in refractory SCI neuropathic pain are warranted.

N-Methyl-d-Aspartate Antagonists

Ketamine and other N-methyl-d-aspartate (NMDA) antagonists have shown promise for relieving neuropathic pain at lower doses than those inducing anesthesia.[81,82]

Positive results have been shown specifically in persons with SCI and chronic central neuropathic pain, including both single-dose infusions[83,84] and a trial that included one infusion of ketamine per day for 7 days as an adjuvant to oral gabapentin.[85] A recent study in 13 patients also suggests that ketamine administration during the acute phase of neuropathic pain symptoms (average time since neuropathic pain onset was 10.3 days) may prevent its development into chronic pain.[86] Although interruption of NMDA receptor mechanisms can produce large reductions in neuropathic pain, the route of administration, dosing scheme, and elimination or reduction of unacceptable side effects still need study.

Antispasticity Agents

Antispasticity agents, such as baclofen, are commonly used to suppress spasticity in patients with SCI and have also been shown to significantly reduce musculoskeletal pain after SCI.[87] However, the effect of IT baclofen on neuropathic pain in SCI has little support,[88] and oral baclofen has not been clinically tested for this indication.

Summary

Pharmacologic agents can be effective for the relief of neuropathic pain in some patients with SCI. The agents with the most evidence of efficacy in this patient group are pregabalin, gabapentin, amitriptyline, tramadol, and duloxetine. Other agents can be tried in refractory cases, as response to treatment and acceptability of side effects vary patient by patient.

NONPHARMACOLOGIC TREATMENT OPTIONS

Patients with SCI and chronic pain are receptive to nonpharmacologic treatments, and most patients have tried at least one type of alternative therapy.[22,44,45] Although there is an evidence basis for some of these interventions for pain in SCI, large randomized controlled trials are infrequent and very few have specifically targeted only patients with neuropathic pain; most studies included persons with SCI and chronic pain of any cause.

The benefit of including these types of therapies in a comprehensive pain management strategy is their general lack of side effects and the ability to combine them with other nonpharmacologic and pharmacologic treatments without significant risk.

Psychological/Cognitive Interventions

The impact that chronic pain has on psychological well-being and overall health and quality of life in individuals with SCI is well documented,[89] and the impact of psychological traits on the maintenance or exacerbation of chronic pain has also been shown.[90,91] It is, therefore, not surprising that interventions aimed at improving coping and cognitive-behavioral management of pain can be successful at reducing pain and increasing general well-being in those patients with chronic pain conditions.[92]

A comprehensive management program for chronic neuropathic pain after SCI should address the potential need for psychological interventions, especially considering the refractory nature of neuropathic pain and the low probability of the complete relief of pain associated with SCI using only pharmacologic agents. Clinical trials for psychological interventions for neuropathic pain in individuals with SCI have been limited, but findings point to a measurable benefit for some patients.

In a small nonrandomized study in persons with disabilities and pain, a cognitive restructuring intervention significantly decreased pain ratings compared with an education control group.[93] Another cognitive-based approach, which was combined with education, stretching, and light exercise, was tested in a sample of persons with SCI and chronic neuropathic pain.[94] Although decreases in pain intensity were not significant at a 12-month follow-up (after the initial 10-week intervention), decreases in depression and increases in the ability to cope with stressors were significantly greater for those in the intervention group compared with those in the control (no intervention) group.[94] A recent multicenter randomized controlled trial of a multidimensional cognitive-behavioral therapy program in persons with SCI-associated neuropathic pain reported significant changes between baseline and the end of treatment for pain intensity, anxiety, pain-related disability, and participation in activities for the test group that were not seen for the control (wait list) group.[95] These differences were not sustained at the 3-month postintervention follow-up, however, suggesting a need for continuous or booster interventions for long-term sustainability for pain management.

The reported results in these studies were based on average changes after treatment pooled across all subjects; therefore, it is not clear what percentage of individuals would be considered responders to psychological and behavioral interventions. In addition, research regarding the patient characteristics that predict success in a pain management program with such interventions would be particularly useful.

Massage

Based on survey studies, the most commonly reported nonpharmacologic treatment tried for pain by those patients with SCI is massage or relaxation therapy, which is reported as effective in most of the patients who have tried it, and conveys, on average, a moderate to substantial reduction in pain.[22,45,96] One study in individuals with neuropathic pain after SCI found that massage therapy twice a week for 6 weeks produced a significant decrease in a pain interference measure at the end of treatment, but it was not sustained at the 2-month posttreatment follow-up.[97] Because long-term use of massage therapy is considered safe and there is some support for its analgesic efficacy, it can be suggested as a complementary or alternative treatment to pharmacologic therapies.

Acupuncture

Although a traditional Eastern therapy, Western medicine has begun to embrace the possibility that acupuncture may confer analgesic effects. In 1997, the National Institutes of Health consensus panel endorsed the use of acupuncture for certain conditions, including pain.[98] Surveys in patients with SCI with persistent pain report that, although many people have tried acupuncture for pain relief (approximately 20%–40%), only a minority of people has found sufficient relief.[45,96] There is only one published prospective study examining the efficacy of acupuncture specifically for post-SCI neuropathic pain.[97] Norrbrink and Lundeberg[97] found that twice-weekly acupuncture sessions over 6 weeks produced a significant reduction in pain compared with baseline levels in 15 subjects with SCI and neuropathic pain, although these improvements were not sustained at a 2-month follow-up visit, and the study did not include a sham control group.[97] An earlier prospective study in subjects with SCI and chronic pain of mixed cause (approximately 50% with probable central neuropathic pain) found that 45% of 22 subjects undergoing 15 acupuncture sessions over 7.5 weeks reported a reduction of at least 2 on the 0 to 10 NRS for pain intensity.[99] This effect was present for 32% of the 22 patients at a 3-month follow-up visit. Post hoc analysis suggested that persons with musculoskeletal pain were more likely to report reductions in pain because of acupuncture than those with neuropathic pain.[99]

Based on limited evidence, it is suggested that acupuncture may be helpful for a minority of patients suffering from neuropathic pain after SCI. Finding a qualified provider, selecting appropriate sites for stimulation, and providing sustained relief of pain may limit its utility for most patients.

Exercise

The effects of regular exercise on health and well-being in the general population are well documented. The impact that regular exercise has on quality of life in persons with SCI has also been reported,[100,101] but the ability of exercise to relieve pain in persons with SCI has not been extensively tested. Studies focusing on shoulder pain in those with SCI have shown reductions in pain when an exercise program has been instituted,[102,103] and a study with nonspecified pain type also reported significant decreases in average pain after a 9-month exercise program.[104] Only one small clinical trial measured the effect of exercise on neuropathic and nociceptive pains (evaluated separately using the ISCIPBD),[105] reporting that neuropathic pain-intensity ratings, as well as nociceptive pain-intensity ratings, were significantly decreased after a 10-week exercise protocol.

Transcutaneous Electrical Nerve Stimulation

Transcutaneous electrical nerve stimulation (TENS) involves the placement of surface electrodes on the skin and the application of electrical current. The placement of the electrodes, typically over the painful area or near the nerves innervating the painful area, as well as the frequency amplitude of the stimulation can be varied to provide maximal effect. Low-frequency (high amplitude) TENS, which is often likened to acupuncture stimulation, works via different, though partially overlapping, mechanisms than high-frequency (low amplitude) TENS.[106] Although TENS has been practiced for several decades, evidence regarding its effectiveness specifically for neuropathic pain is relatively recent. The guidelines on neurostimulation therapy for neuropathic pain in general, published in 2007, concluded that low-frequency TENS had some efficacy for reducing neuropathic pain and that high-frequency TENS was "possibly better than placebo."[106]

Two studies have been published specifically evaluating the effect of TENS for alleviating neuropathic pain in persons with SCI. A study by Norrbrink[107] compared the effectiveness of high- and low-frequency TENS when delivered 3 times per day for 2 weeks and found no significant differences in pain intensity before versus after treatment for either frequency, although approximately 25% of subjects requested to continue TENS treatment after the study was concluded. A more recent study by Celik and colleagues[108] reported significant decreases in pain for subjects assigned to a low-frequency TENS group (once a day for 10 days) compared with those assigned to the sham group. Differences in the results of the 2 studies may be caused by differences in the recency of injury in the 2 samples ($\leq$27 months after injury in the Celik[108] study; average of 6.8 years after injury in the Norrbrink[107] study).

Transcranial Stimulation

A recent review of noninvasive electrical and magnetic neural stimulation in persons with SCI and chronic pain concluded that, although more study is clearly needed, noninvasive transcranial stimulation techniques provide a potentially effective treatment strategy that may be particularly useful for pains with neuropathic characteristics (eg, presence of dysesthesias and allodynia and location of pain in the lower limbs).[109] A small number of studies in the literature have specifically tested patients with SCI and neuropathic pain using controlled trials of transcranial stimulation and have found significant, although somewhat modest, effects,[110,111] though one recent study in a small sample (n = 17) did not show significant reductions in pain compared with sham stimulation.[112] Because of its noninvasive nature, transcranial stimulation may be an option for some patients, although the duration of the effects and side effects, including headaches and cognitive effects, may limit its use.

Motor Cortex Stimulation

Motor cortex stimulation is an invasive technique that consists of using implanted epidural electrodes placed over the motor cortex to cyclically stimulate the area. This treatment technique is reserved for those who have failed all traditional treatments and still have high levels of pain. Much of the evidence for motor cortex stimulation involves case series in patients with central poststroke pain, which indicate that approximately 50% to 60% of these patients obtain relief.[106] A case study reported by Tani and colleagues[113] reported significant relief of intractable pain in a patient with SCI with 30-minute stimulation periods 3 to 4 times a day. A case series of 31 patients with neuropathic pain of central origin found 40% or more pain relief in 52% of subjects during an average 49-month follow-up period, along with a decrease in analgesic drug intake in approximately 55% of subjects.[114] Similarly, an earlier case series[115] reported 40% or more pain relief over a 27-month follow-up period in approximately 75% of patients with either central pain or trigeminal pain. However, only 2 of 6 patients with SCI-related pain in these 2 studies had successful outcomes at follow-up.[114–116]

Motor cortex stimulation has been advocated as a potentially valuable treatment option for intractable pain in SCI because it has shown some efficacy and the risk of medical complications (eg, seizure, wound infection) is relatively small.[106,117]

Deep Brain Stimulation

Stimulation of thalamic nuclei, periaqueductal or periventricular gray, and the internal capsule have been targeted for stimulation to relieve pain in persons with SCI.[116] Most studies of deep brain stimulation (DBS) are case series or retrospective analyses without proper controls or randomization; but, given the nature of this invasive technique, such controlled blinded studies would be unethical. Evidence for DBS is stronger for nociceptive pain, but neuropathic pain caused by peripheral lesions has also been effectively treated by DBS. Evidence for the effectiveness of DBS in the treatment of other types of pain is equivocal.[106] Several of the published trials with DBS have included some patients with chronic neuropathic pain caused by SCI; although half of these patients have experienced short-term reductions in pain, the results from long-term follow-up (between 6 and 80 months, depending on the study) have shown success in only 16% of patients with SCI.[116]

Because of the invasive nature of DBS and weak evidence of long-term efficacy in persons with chronic pain after SCI, it is currently not recommended as a treatment in this patient population.[18,116] Major adverse events include infections and intracranial hemorrhages and can require additional surgery and removal of stimulators.[116,118]

Spinal Cord Stimulation

Spinal cord stimulation (SCS) techniques involve the placement of electrodes into the epidural space around the spine. Placement of the electrodes must be in the appropriate location so that stimulation evokes paresthesias that cover the area where pain is reported. Although the exact mechanisms underlying SCS's effects are not known, it is generally thought that gate control–like mechanisms,[119] including activation of the dorsal columns, play a major role and that, for SCS to be successful, patients should have some sparing of the dorsal columns.[106,120] SCS has been recommended, albeit weakly to moderately, for use in patients with failed back surgery syndrome[106,121,122] when other less-invasive options have been ineffective. Some evidence also supports its use for complex regional pain syndrome (CRPS) type I,[106,121,122] and most suggest that success is generally better in patients with peripheral types of neuropathic pain compared with those with central neuropathic pain syndromes.[106] A recent case series report, however, found that approximately half of their patients with poststroke central pain had 30% or more pain reduction during a stimulation trial and that 6 of 9 patients with permanently implanted SCS devices rated their condition as *much improved* at the follow-up period (average 28 months).[123]

Published trials examining the efficacy of SCS in persons with intractable neuropathic pain after SCI provide limited data. One published report in 127 patients with various central pain conditions found that those with complete SCI (n = 11) were very unlikely to benefit from SCS (fair relief of pain in 20%), but those with incomplete SCI (n = 24) were a bit more likely to benefit from SCI (27% good relief and 14% fair relief).[124] Similarly, Cioni and colleagues[125] reported that only 4 patients (of an initial 35) had long-term substantial relief (mean follow-up of 37 months); all of these patients had incomplete SCIs.

Patients who may be candidates for permanent implantation of an SCS undergo a trial period with a temporarily implanted device. Success with the temporary implant is thought to predict those who will benefit from a permanently implanted SCS; but most patients do not find continued efficacy past 1 year, and SCS has not been recommended for those with complete SCIs.[126] Recently, a screening tool for guidance regarding the selection of patients that may gain the most benefit from SCS has been published by an international group of pain specialists.[127]

COMBINATION THERAPIES

Because patients with SCI may be taking several medications for various conditions, great care is needed to assess the potential for adverse events caused by interactions among pharmacologic agents. However, as stated in the introduction, many people with SCI suffer from more than one type of pain, which likely involves many different mechanisms that can best be targeted with combination therapies. Additionally, most treatments for neuropathic pain after SCI offer only partial relief; increases in the dose may be precluded by adverse side effects, so the introduction of a new treatment, which works via different mechanisms within the neuropathic pain pathway, can improve outcomes.

Combinations of gabapentin or pregabalin with opioids have been assessed in patients with postherpetic or diabetic neuropathic pain types. Published trials indicate an improvement in pain relief at lower doses when these drug classes have been combined compared with their effectiveness when administered separately.[64] The combination of gabapentin with nortriptyline in the same patient populations have shown similar results: greater decreases in pain for combination therapy than when either drug was administered alone.[128] One study in patients with SCI-related neuropathic pain evaluated the effect of a daily infusion of ketamine and oral gabapentin and found significant relief with this combination therapy.[85] However, results were not compared with the administration of the drugs separately, so conclusions regarding the enhanced efficacy of this combination cannot be made.

It has been suggested that patients who tolerate and find some relief from each of the drugs separately be offered a combination of the drugs at lower dosages to further enhance pain relief without additional side effects.[128] However, a recent Cochrane review concluded that side effects from combination therapies generally produced a greater amount of subject dropout compared with when drugs are administered separately.[129] The guidelines from the European Federation of Neurologic Societies in 2010 endorsed the use of combinations of gabapentin with opioids and gabapentin with antidepressants for the treatment of neuropathic pain in those patients for whom these agents were not sufficient when delivered alone.[42]

SURGICAL TREATMENT OPTIONS

Surgical techniques required to address structural problems of the vertebral column in patients with acute SCI may be necessary to avoid the development of pain conditions caused by nerve compression. Surgical procedures, such as ablation of the nerve tracts implicated in pain, have also been used in patients with chronic SCI who have already developed neuropathic pain. Although several reports of these types of procedures exist in the literature, they are frequently lacking in details regarding characteristics of the SCI, including completeness and level of injury, and type of pain.[130] Because of the invasive and irreversible nature of this type of treatment, controlled, randomized, and blinded trials do not exist.

The dorsal root entry zone (DREZ) lesion is performed by sectioning the tip of the dorsal horn at the area of entry to the spinal column at or above the level of the SCI. By ablating this area, hyperactive neurons that may be responsible for pain are eliminated. Some prospective studies have documented high levels of sustained pain reduction in approximately 50% of patients on whom this procedure was performed.[123,130] Such positive results are limited to those with at-level neuropathic pain localized to a small band of dermatomes around the level of injury, whereas DREZ lesions have produced successes in only a minority of patients with more diffuse pain related to central or below-level neuropathic pain.[18,130–132] Complications from these procedures include cerebrospinal fluid leaks, epidural hematoma, and potential increase in weakness below the level of the lesion.[131]

Reports of cordotomy, cordectomy, and cordomyelotomy for pain related to SCI are present in the literature; but details are lacking, and these procedures are generally not recommended.[121,133]

EVALUATION OF OUTCOME

The use of a selection of the tools presented earlier ("Tools for Diagnosis and Evaluation of Neuropathic Pain" and in **Table 1**) can assist with the evaluation of outcomes after an intervention. Having standardized and validated assessments available at follow-up to compare with baseline values promotes a less biased assessment of treatment efficacy. In addition to the recommendations discussed earlier, the PGIC, a record of the amount of other analgesics, and an inquiry regarding side effects and tolerability are helpful to understand the success of an intervention.

The PGIC is recommended for use in clinical trials of analgesics[35] and is typically composed of one question regarding patients' perception of how much improved their condition is since the start of a treatment. There are 7 options for response, ranging from *very much improved* to *very much worse*. This type of question allows patients to weigh the amount of pain relief they are obtaining against the tolerability of side effects and to assess whether the treatment has made a positive, negative, or neutral contribution to their function and quality of life. Using a graded, Likert-type scale to assess the response to treatment assists patients and the provider with a gauge of the success of the treatment strategy and opens the dialogue regarding whether changes should be made to improve the pain management program.

SUMMARY

Many patients with neuropathic pain after SCI are currently unable to find satisfactory management for their pain. It has been repeatedly acknowledged that a multifaceted approach that combines therapies aimed at correcting biologic mechanisms with therapies that engage coping mechanisms and improves functional outcomes is the preferred pain management model.[11,94] However, such comprehensive approaches are frequently cost prohibitive because of a lack of insurance coverage/reimbursement and are largely untested.

When initially evaluating patients with a chronic pain condition, multiple factors should be considered, and documented responses to questionnaires and other assessments will be helpful to compare with responses at follow-up. Because patients with SCI commonly have more than one type of pain, clinical evaluation should include a detailed evaluation of all pain complaints in order to determine whether multiple approaches to pain relief may be necessary.

Some pharmacologic options exist that are helpful in a subset of patients, including pregabalin and gabapentin and, to a lesser extent, amitriptyline and duloxetine. Recommendations for other approaches, if these agents fail, are limited because of insufficient evidence in the literature, which lacks high-quality studies specifically in patients with neuropathic pain caused by SCI. Based on the patient's situation and clinical judgment, the use of opioids, cannabinoids, and more invasive interventions (eg, transcranial stimulation, SCS) may be proposed. Patients should be encouraged to embark on cognitive-behavioral therapies, massage, acupuncture, or exercise for pain management, as these approaches are endorsed by many patients with SCI and chronic pain themselves, based on survey studies in the literature.

REFERENCES

1. Störmer S, Gerner HJ, Grüninger W, et al. Chronic pain/dysaesthesiae in spinal cord injury patients: results of a multicentre study. Spinal Cord 1997;35:446–55.
2. Demirel G, Yllmaz H, Gençosmanoğlu B, et al. Pain following spinal cord injury. Spinal Cord 1998;36:25–8.
3. Turner JA, Cardenas DD. Chronic pain problems in individuals with spinal cord injuries. Semin Clin Neuropsychiatry 1999;4:186–94.
4. Widerström-Noga EG, Felipe-Cuervo E, Broton JG, et al. Perceived difficulty in dealing with consequences of spinal cord injury. Arch Phys Med Rehabil 1999; 80:580–6.
5. Finnerup NB, Johannesen IL, Sindrup SH, et al. Pain and dysesthesia in patients with spinal cord injury: a postal survey. Spinal Cord 2001;39:256–62.
6. Siddall PJ, McClelland JM, Rutkowski SB, et al. A longitudinal study of the prevalence and characteristics of pain in the first 5 years following spinal cord injury. Pain 2003;103:249–57.
7. Cruz-Almeida Y, Martinez-Arizala A, Widerström-Noga EG. Chronicity of pain associated with spinal cord injury: a longitudinal analysis. J Rehabil Res Dev 2005;42:585–94.
8. Cardenas DD, Felix ER. Pain after spinal cord injury: a review of classification, treatment approaches, and treatment assessment. PM R 2009;1(12):1077–90.
9. Cardenas DD, Turner JA, Warms CA, et al. Classification of chronic pain associated with spinal cord injuries. Arch Phys Med Rehabil 2002;83:1708–14.
10. Werhagen L, Budh CN, Hultling C, et al. Neuropathic pain after traumatic spinal cord injury–relations to gender, spinal level, completeness, and age at the time of injury. Spinal Cord 2004;42:665–73.

11. Salle JY, Ginies P, Perrouin-Verbe B, et al. Pain management: what's the more efficient model? Ann Phys Rehabil Med 2009;52(2):203–9.
12. Turk DC, Dworkin RH, Allen RR, et al. Core outcome domains for chronic pain clinical trials: IMMPACT recommendations. Pain 2003;106:337–45.
13. Calmels P, Mick G, Perrouin-Verbe B, et al, SOFMER (French Society for Physical Medicine and Rehabilitation). Neuropathic pain in spinal cord injury: identification, classification, evaluation. Ann Phys Rehabil Med 2009;52:83–102.
14. Haanpaa M, Attal N, Backonja M, et al. NeuPSIG guidelines on neuropathic pain assessment. Pain 2011;152(1):14–27.
15. Treede RD, Jensen TS, Campbell JN, et al. Neuropathic pain: redefinition and a grading system for clinical and research purposes. Neurology 2008;70:1630–5.
16. Finnerup NB, Sorensen L, Biering-Sorensen F, et al. Segmental hypersensitivity and spinothalamic function in spinal cord injury pain. Exp Neurol 2007;207:139–49.
17. Finnerup NB. Predictors of spinal cord injury neuropathic pain: the role of QST. Top Spinal Cord Inj Rehabil 2007;13:35–42.
18. Finnerup NB, Baastrup C. SCI pain: mechanisms and management. Curr Pain Headache Rep 2012;16:207–16.
19. Backonja MM, Attal N, Baron R, et al. Value of quantitative sensory testing in neurological and pain disorders: NeuPSIG consensus. Pain 2013;154:1807–19.
20. Felix ER, Cruz-Almeida Y, Widerström-Noga EG. Chronic pain after spinal cord injury: what characteristics make some pains more disturbing than others? J Rehabil Res Dev 2007;44:703–16.
21. Jensen MP, Widerström-Noga E, Richards JS, et al. Reliability and validity of the international spinal cord injury basic pain data set items as self-report measures. Spinal Cord 2010;48:230–8.
22. Heutink M, Post MW, Wollaars MM, et al. Chronic spinal cord injury pain: pharmacological and non-pharmacological treatments and treatment effectiveness. Disabil Rehabil 2011;33(5):433–40.
23. Widerström-Noga E, Biering-Sørensen F, Bryce T, et al. The international SCI pain basic data set. Spinal Cord 2008;86:818–23.
24. Widerstrom-Noga E, Biering-Sorensen F, Bryce T, et al. The International Spinal Cord Injury Pain Basic Data Set (version 2.0). Spinal Cord 2014;52:282–6.
25. Bryce TN, Biering-Sørensen F, Finnerup NB, et al. International SCI pain classification: part I. Background and description. Spinal Cord 2012;50:413–7.
26. Bryce TN, Biering-Sørensen F, Finnerup NB, et al. International Spinal Cord Injury Pain (ISCIP) classification: part 2. Initial validation using vignettes. Spinal Cord 2012;50:404–12.
27. Jensen TS, Baron R, Haanpää M, et al. A new definition of neuropathic pain. Pain 2011;152:2204–5.
28. Haanpää ML, Backonja MM, Bennett MI, et al. Assessment of neuropathic pain in primary care. Am J Med 2009;122(Suppl 10):S13–21.
29. Bennett M. The LANSS Pain Scale: the Leeds assessment of neuropathic symptoms and signs. Pain 2001;92:147–57.
30. Bouhassira D, Attal N, Alchaar H, et al. Comparison of pain syndromes associated with nervous or somatic lesions and development of a new neuropathic pain diagnostic questionnaire (DN4). Pain 2005;114:29–36.
31. Kirshblum SC, Burns SP, Biering-Sorensen F, et al. International standards for neurological classification of spinal cord injury (revised 2011). J Spinal Cord Med 2011;34:535–46.

32. Galer BS, Jensen MP. Development and preliminary validation of a pain measure specific to neuropathic pain: the Neuropathic Pain Scale. Neurology 1997;48:332–8.

33. Bouhassira D, Attal N, Fermanian J, et al. Development and validation of the Neuropathic Pain Symptom Inventory. Pain 2004;108:248–57.

34. Cleeland CS, Ryan KM. Pain assessment: global use of the Brief Pain Inventory. Ann Acad Med Singap 1994;23:129–38.

35. Dworkin RH, Turk DC, Farrar JT, et al, IMMPACT. Core outcome measures for chronic pain clinical trials: IMMPACT recommendations. Pain 2005;113:9–19.

36. Celestin J, Edwards RR, Jamison RN. Pretreatment psychosocial variables as predictors of outcomes following lumbar surgery and spinal cord stimulation: a systematic review and literature synthesis. Pain Med 2009;10:639–53.

37. de Rooij A, Roorda LD, Otten RH, et al. Predictors of multidisciplinary treatment outcome in fibromyalgia: a systematic review. Disabil Rehabil 2013;35:437–49.

38. Beck AT, Ward CH, Mendelson M, et al. An inventory for measuring depression. Arch Gen Psychiatry 1961;4:561–71.

39. Spielberger CD, Gorsuch RL, Lushene SH. Manual for the State-Trait Anxiety Inventory. Palo Alto, CA: Consulting Psychologist Press; 1970.

40. Zigmond AS, Snaith RP. The hospital anxiety and depression scale. Acta Psychiatr Scand 1983;67:361–70.

41. Sullivan MJ, Bishop SR, Pivik J. The pain catastrophizing scale: development and validation. Psychol Assess 1995;7:524–32.

42. Attal N, Cruccu G, Baron R, et al. EFNS guidelines on the pharmacological treatment of neuropathic pain: 2010 revision. Eur J Neurol 2010;17(9):1113–23.

43. Warms CA, Turner JA, Marshall HM, et al. Treatments for chronic pain associated with spinal cord injuries: many are tried, few are helpful. Clin J Pain 2002;18:154–63.

44. Widerström-Noga EG, Turk DC. Types and effectiveness of treatments used by people with chronic pain associated with spinal cord injuries: influence of pain and psychosocial characteristics. Spinal Cord 2003;41(11):600–9.

45. Cardenas DD, Jensen MP. Treatments for chronic pain in persons with spinal cord injury: a survey study. J Spinal Cord Med 2006;29:109–17.

46. Attal N, Mazaltarine G, Perrouin-Verbe B, et al. Chronic neuropathic pain management in spinal cord injury patient. What is the efficacy of pharmacological treatments with general mode of administration? (oral, transdermal, intravenous). Ann Phys Rehabil Med 2009;52(2):124–41.

47. Siddall PJ, Middleton JW. A proposed algorithm for the management of pain following spinal cord injury. Spinal Cord 2006;44(2):67–77.

48. Siddall PJ, Cousins MJ, Otte A, et al. Pregabalin in central neuropathic pain associated with spinal cord injury: a placebo-controlled trial. Neurology 2006; 67:1792–800.

49. Cardenas DD, Nieshoff EC, Suda K, et al. A randomized trial of pregabalin in patients with neuropathic pain due to spinal cord injury. Neurology 2013;80:533–9.

50. Vranken JH, Dijkgraaf MG, Kruis MR, et al. Pregabalin in patients with central neuropathic pain: a randomized, double-blind, placebo-controlled trial of a flexible-dose regimen. Pain 2008;136:150–7.

51. Dalal K, Felix ER, Cardenas DD. Pregabalin for the management of neuropathic pain in spinal cord injury. Pain Manag 2013;3(5):359–67.

52. Levendoglu F, Ogün CO, Ozerbil O, et al. Gabapentin is a first line drug for the treatment of neuropathic pain in spinal cord injury. Spine (Phila Pa 1976) 2004; 29:743–51.

53. Ahn SH, Park HW, Lee BS, et al. Gabapentin effect on neuropathic pain compared among patients with spinal cord injury and different durations of symptoms. Spine (Phila Pa 1976) 2003;28:341–7.
54. Tai Q, Kirshblum S, Chen B, et al. Gabapentin in the treatment of neuropathic pain after spinal cord injury: a prospective, randomized, double-blind, cross-over trial. J Spinal Cord Med 2002;25:100–5.
55. To TP, Lim TC, Hill ST, et al. Gabapentin for neuropathic pain following spinal cord injury. Spinal Cord 2002;40:282–5.
56. Putzke JD, Richards JS, Kezar L, et al. Long-term use of gabapentin for treatment of pain after traumatic spinal cord injury. Clin J Pain 2002;18:116–21.
57. Rintala DH, Holmes SA, Courtade D, et al. Comparison of the effectiveness of amitriptyline and gabapentin on chronic neuropathic pain in persons with spinal cord injury. Arch Phys Med Rehabil 2007;88:1547–60.
58. Finnerup NB, Grydehøj J, Bing J, et al. Levetiracetam in spinal cord injury pain: a randomized controlled trial. Spinal Cord 2009;47:861–7.
59. Drewes AM, Andreasen A, Poulsen LH. Valproate for treatment of chronic central pain after spinal cord injury. A double-blind cross-over study. Paraplegia 1994;32:565–9.
60. Finnerup NB, Sindrup SH, Bach FW, et al. Lamotrigine in spinal cord injury pain: a randomized controlled trial. Pain 2002;96:375–83.
61. Salinas FA, Lugo LH, García HI. Efficacy of early treatment with carbamazepine in prevention of neuropathic pain in patients with spinal cord injury. Am J Phys Med Rehabil 2012;91:1020–7.
62. Saarto T, Wiffen P. Antidepressants for neuropathic pain: a Cochrane review. J Neurol Neurosurg Psychiatry 2010;81:1372–3.
63. Moore RA, Derry S, Aldington D, et al. Amitriptyline for neuropathic pain and fibromyalgia in adults. Cochrane Database Syst Rev 2012;(12):CD008242.
64. Dworkin RH, O'Connor AB, Audette J, et al. Recommendations for pharmacological management of neuropathic pain; an overview and literature update. Mayo Clin Proc 2010;85(Suppl 3):S3–14.
65. Cardenas DD, Warms CA, Turner JA, et al. Efficacy of amitriptyline for relief of pain in spinal cord injury: results of a randomized controlled trial. Pain 2002; 96:365–73.
66. Kajdasz DK, Iyengar S, Desaiah D, et al. Duloxetine for the management of diabetic peripheral neuropathic pain: evidence-based findings from post hoc analysis of three multicenter, randomized, double-blind, placebo-controlled, parallel-group studies. Clin Ther 2007;29(Suppl):2536–46.
67. Vranken JH, Hollmann MW, van der Veegt MH, et al. Duloxetine in patients with central neuropathic pain caused by spinal cord injury or stroke: a randomized, double-blind, placebo-controlled trial. Pain 2011;152(2):267–73.
68. Kadiroglu AK, Sit D, Kayabasi H, et al. The effect of venlafaxine HCl on painful peripheral diabetic neuropathy in patients with type 2 diabetes mellitus. J Diabetes Complications 2008;22:241–5.
69. Sindrup SH, Bach FW, Madsen C, et al. Venlafaxine versus imipramine in painful polyneuropathy: a randomized, controlled trial. Neurology 2003; 60(8):1284–9.
70. Norrbrink C, Lundeberg T. Tramadol in neuropathic pain after spinal cord injury: a randomized, double-blind, placebo-controlled trial. Clin J Pain 2009;25(3): 177–84.
71. Hollingshead J, Dühmke RM, Cornblath DR. Tramadol for neuropathic pain. Cochrane Database Syst Rev 2006;(3):CD003726.

72. Barrera-Chacon JM, Mendez-Suarez JL, Jauregui-Abrisqueta ML, et al. Oxycodone improves pain control and quality of life in anticonvulsant-pretreated spinal cord-injured patients with neuropathic pain. Spinal Cord 2011;49(1):36–42.

73. Attal N, Guirimand F, Brasseur L, et al. Effects of IV morphine in central pain: a randomized placebo-controlled study. Neurology 2002;58:554–63.

74. Siddall PJ, Molloy AR, Walker S, et al. The efficacy of intrathecal morphine and clonidine in the treatment of pain after spinal cord injury. Anesth Analg 2000;91: 1493–8.

75. Bensmail D, Ecoffey C, Ventura M, et al. Chronic neuropathic pain in patients with spinal cord injury. What is the efficacy of regional interventions? Sympathetic blocks, nerve blocks and intrathecal drugs. Ann Phys Rehabil Med 2009;52(2):142–8.

76. Rintala DH, Fiess RN, Tan G, et al. Effect of dronabinol on central neuropathic pain after spinal cord injury: a pilot study. Am J Phys Med Rehabil 2010;89: 840–8.

77. Wilsey B, Marotte T, Tsodikov A, et al. A randomized, placebo-controlled, cross-over trial of cannabis cigarettes in neuropathic pain. J Pain 2008;9(6):506–21.

78. Ware MA, Wang T, Shapiro S, et al. Smoked cannabis for chronic neuropathic pain: a randomized controlled trial. CMAJ 2010;182(14):E694–701.

79. Wilsey B, Marcotte T, Deutsch R, et al. Low-dose vaporized cannabis significantly improves neuropathic pain. J Pain 2013;14(2):136–48.

80. Langford RM, Mares J, Novotna A, et al. A double-blind, randomized, placebo-controlled, parallel-group study of THC/CBD oromucosal spray in combination with the existing treatment regimen, in the relief of central neuropathic pain in patients with multiple sclerosis. J Neurol 2013;260(4):984–97.

81. Backonja M, Arndt G, Gombar KA, et al. Response of chronic neuropathic pain syndromes to ketamine: a preliminary study. Pain 1994;56:51–7.

82. Niesters M, Dahan A. Pharmacokinetic and pharmacodynamic considerations for NMDA receptor antagonists in the treatment of chronic neuropathic pain. Expert Opin Drug Metab Toxicol 2012;8:1409–17.

83. Eide PK, Stubhaug A, Stenehjem AE. Central dysesthesia pain after traumatic spinal cord injury is dependent on N-methyl-d-aspartate receptor activation. Neurosurgery 1995;37(6):1080–7.

84. Kvarnstrom A, Karlsten R, Quiding H, et al. The analgesic effect of intravenous ketamine and lidocaine on pain after spinal cord injury. Acta Anaesthesiol Scand 2004;48(4):498–506.

85. Amr YM. Multi-day low dose ketamine infusion as adjuvant to oral gabapentin in spinal cord injury related chronic pain: a prospective, randomized, double blind trial. Pain Physician 2010;13(3):245–9.

86. Kim K, Mishina M, Kukubo R, et al. Ketamine for acute neuropathic pain in patients with spinal cord injury. J Clin Neurosci 2013;20:804–7.

87. Loubser PG, Akman NM. Effects of intrathecal baclofen on chronic spinal cord injury pain. J Pain Symptom Manage 1996;12:241–7.

88. Teasell RW, Mehta S, Aubut JA, et al. A systematic review of pharmacologic treatments of pain after spinal cord injury. Arch Phys Med Rehabil 2010;91: 816–31.

89. Finnerup NB. Pain in patients with spinal cord injury. Pain 2013;154(Suppl 1): S71–6.

90. Widerström-Noga EG, Felix ER, Cruz-Almeida Y, et al. Psychosocial subgroups in persons with spinal cord injuries and chronic pain. Arch Phys Med Rehabil 2007;88:1628–35.

91. Wollaars MM, Post MW, van Asbeck FW, et al. Spinal cord injury pain: the influence of psychologic factors and impact on quality of life. Clin J Pain 2007;23: 383–91.

92. Gault D, Morel-Fatio M, Albert T, et al. Chronic neuropathic pain of spinal cord injury what is the effectiveness of psychocomportemental management? Ann Phys Rehabil Med 2009;52(2):167–72.

93. Ehde DM, Jensen M. Feasibility of a cognitive restructuring intervention for treatment of chronic pain in persons with disabilities. Rehabil Psychol 2004;49: 254–8.

94. Norrbrink Budh C, Kowalski J, Lundeberg T. A comprehensive pain management programme comprising educational, cognitive and behavioural interventions for neuropathic pain following spinal cord injury. J Rehabil Med 2006;38: 172–80.

95. Heutink M, Post MW, Bongers-Janssen HM, et al. The CONECSI trial: results of a randomized controlled trial of a multidisciplinary cognitive behavioral program for coping with chronic neuropathic pain after spinal cord injury. Pain 2012; 153:120–8.

96. Norrbrink Budh C, Lundeberg T. Non-pharmacological pain-relieving therapies in individuals with spinal cord injury: a patient perspective. Complement Ther Med 2004;12:189–97.

97. Norrbrink C, Lundeberg T. Acupuncture and massage therapy for neuropathic pain following spinal cord injury: an exploratory study. Acupunct Med 2011; 29:108–15.

98. NIH consensus developmental panel on acupuncture. JAMA 1998;280: 1518–24.

99. Nayak S, Shiflett SC, Schoenberger NE, et al. Is acupuncture effective in treating chronic pain after spinal cord injury? Arch Phys Med Rehabil 2001;82:1578–86.

100. Stotts KM. Health maintenance: paraplegic athletes and nonathletes. Arch Phys Med Rehabil 1986;67:109–14.

101. Devillard X, Rimaud D, Roche F, et al. Effects of training programs for spinal cord injury. Ann Readapt Med Phys 2007;50:490–8, 480–9.

102. Curtis KA, Tyner TM, Zachary L, et al. Effect of a standard exercise protocol on shoulder pain in long-term wheelchair users. Spinal Cord 1999;37:421–9.

103. Nawoczenski DA, Ritter-Soronen JM, Wilson CM, et al. Clinical trial of exercise for shoulder pain in chronic spinal injury. Phys Ther 2006;86:1604–18.

104. Hicks AL, Martin KA, Ditor DS, et al. Long-term exercise training in persons with spinal cord injury: effects on strength, arm ergometry performance and psychological well-being. Spinal Cord 2003;41:34–43.

105. Norrbrink C, Lindberg T, Wahman K, et al. Effects of an exercise programme on musculoskeletal and neuropathic pain after spinal cord injury–results from a seated double-poling ergometer study. Spinal Cord 2012;50(6):457–61.

106. Cruccu G, Aziz TZ, Garcia-Larrea L, et al. EFNS guidelines on neurostimulation therapy for neuropathic pain. Eur J Neurol 2007;14:952–70.

107. Norrbrink C. Transcutaneous electrical nerve stimulation for treatment of spinal cord injury neuropathic pain. J Rehabil Res Dev 2009;46(1):85–93.

108. Celik EC, Erhan B, Cunduz B, et al. The effect of low-frequency TENS in the treatment of neuropathic pain in patients with spinal cord injury. Spinal Cord 2013;51(4):334–7.

109. Moreno-Duarte I, Morse LR, Alam M, et al. Targeted therapies using electrical and magnetic neural stimulation for the treatment of chronic pain in spinal cord injury. Neuroimage 2014;85(Pt 3):1003–13.

110. Capel ID, Dorrell HM, Spencer EP, et al. The amelioration of the suffering associated with spinal cord injury with subperception transcranial electrical stimulation. Spinal Cord 2003;41:109–17.
111. Tan G, Rintala DH, Thornby JI, et al. Using cranial electrotherapy stimulation to treat pain associated with spinal cord injury. J Rehabil Res Dev 2006;43: 461–74.
112. Yılmaz B, Kesikburun S, Yas Ar E, et al. The effect of repetitive transcranial magnetic stimulation on refractory neuropathic pain in spinal cord injury. J Spinal Cord Med 2013. [Epub ahead of print].
113. Tani N, Saitoh Y, Hirata M, et al. Bilateral cortical stimulation for deafferentation pain after spinal cord injury. Case report. J Neurosurg 2004;101(4):687–9.
114. Nuti C, Peyron R, Garcia-Larrea L, et al. Motor cortex stimulation for refractory neuropathic pain: four year outcome and predictors of efficacy. Pain 2005; 118(1–2):43–52.
115. Nguyen JP, Lefaucheur JP, Cecq P, et al. Chronic motor cortex stimulation in the treatment of central and neuropathic pain. Correlations between clinical, electrophysiological and anatomical data. Pain 1999;82(3):245–51.
116. Previnaire JG, Nguyen JP, Perroiun-Verbe B, et al. Chronic neuropathic pain in spinal cord injury: efficiency of deep brain and motor cortex stimulation therapies for neuropathic pain in spinal cord injury patients. Ann Phys Rehabil Med 2009;52:188–93.
117. Nardone R, Höller Y, Leis S, et al. Invasive and non-invasive brain stimulation for treatment of neuropathic pain in patients with spinal cord injury: a review. J Spinal Cord Med 2014;37:19–31.
118. Levy RM, Lamb S, Adams JE. Treatment of chronic pain by deep brain stimulation: long term follow-up and review of the literature. Neurosurgery 1987;21: 885–93.
119. Melzack R, Wall PD. Pain mechanisms: a new theory. Science 1965;150:971–9.
120. Son BC, Kim DR, Lee SW, et al. Factors associated with the success of trial spinal cord stimulation in patients with chronic pain from failed back surgery syndrome. J Korean Neurosurg Soc 2013;54(6):501–6.
121. Dworkin RH, O'Connor AB, Kent J, et al. Interventional management of neuropathic pain: NeuPSIG recommendations. Pain 2013;154(11):2249–61.
122. Mailis A, Taenzer P. Evidence-based guideline for neuropathic pain interventional treatments: spinal cord stimulation, intravenous infusions, epidural injections and nerve blocks. Pain Res Manag 2012;17(3):150–8.
123. Aly MM, Saitoh Y, Hosomi K, et al. Spinal cord stimulation for central poststroke pain. Neurosurgery 2010;67(3 Suppl Operative):ons206–12.
124. Tasker RR, DeCarvalho GT, Dolan EJ. Intractable pain of spinal cord origin: clinical features and implication for surgery. J Neurosurg 1992;77(3):373–8.
125. Cioni B, Meglio M, Pentimalli L, et al. Spinal cord stimulation in the treatment of paraplegic pain. J Neurosurg 1995;82:35–9.
126. Lagauche D, Facione J, Albert T, et al. The chronic neuropathic pain of spinal cord injury: which efficiency of neuropathic stimulation? Ann Phys Rehabil Med 2009;52(2):182–7.
127. Baron R, Backonia MM, Eldridge P, et al. Refractory Chronic Pain Screening Tool (RCPST): a feasibility study to assess practicality and validity of identifying potential neurostimulation candidates. Pain Med 2014;15(2):281–91.
128. Gilron I, Baily JM, Tu D, et al. Nortriptyline and gabapentin, alone and in combination for neuropathic pain: a double-blind, randomized controlled crossover trial. Lancet 2009;374(9697):1252–61.

129. Chaparro LE, Wiffen PJ, Moore RA, et al. Combination pharmacotherapy for the treatment of neuropathic pain in adults. Cochrane Database Syst Rev 2012;(7):CD008943.
130. Robert R, Perrouin-Verbe B, Albert T, et al. Chronic neuropathic pain in spinal cord injured patients: what is the effectiveness of surgical treatments excluding central neurostimulations? Ann Phys Rehabil Med 2009;52(2):194–202.
131. Friedman AH, Nashold BS Jr. DREZ lesions for relief of pain related to spinal cord injury. J Neurosurg 1986;65:465–9.
132. Falci S, Best L, Bayles R, et al. Dorsal root entry zone microcoagulation for spinal cord injury-related central pain: operative intramedullary electrophysiological guidance and clinical outcome. J Neurosurg 2002;97(Suppl 2):193–200.
133. Siddall PJ. Management of neuropathic pain following spinal cord injury: now and in the future. Spinal Cord 2009;47(5):352–9.
134. IASP Task Force on Taxonomy. Part III: pain terms, a current list with definitions and notes on usage. In: Merskey H, Bogduk N, editors. Classification of chronic pain. 2nd edition. Seattle (WA): IASP Press; 1994. p. 209–14 Updated, 2012. Available at: https://www.iasp-pain.org/Education/Content.aspx?ItemNumber=1698.
135. Krause SJ, Backonja MM. Development of a neuropathic pain questionnaire. Clin J Pain 2003;19:306–14.
136. Freynhagen R, Baron R, Gockel U, et al. painDETECT: a new screening questionnaire to identify neuropathic components in patients with back pain. Curr Med Res Opin 2006;22:1911–20.
137. Portenoy R. Development and testing of a neuropathic pain screening questionnaire: ID Pain. Curr Med Res Opin 2006;22:1555–65.
138. Raichle KA, Osborne TL, Jensen MP, et al. The reliability and validity of pain interference measures in persons with spinal cord injury. J Pain 2006;7:179–86.
139. Kerns RD, Turk DC, Rudy TE. The West Haven-Yale Multidimensional Pain Inventory (WHYMPI). Pain 1985;23:345–56.
140. Widerström-Noga EG, Cruz-Almeida Y, Martinez-Arizala A, et al. Internal consistency, stability, and validity of the spinal cord injury version of the Multidimensional Pain Inventory. Arch Phys Med Rehabil 2006;87:516–23.

Reducing Cardiometabolic Disease in Spinal Cord Injury

Jochen Kressler, PhD[a,b], Rachel E. Cowan, PhD[a,b],
Gregory E. Bigford, PhD[a,b], Mark S. Nash, PhD[a,b,c],*

KEYWORDS

- Diet • Exercise • Behavioral modification • Drug therapy
- Cardiometabolic syndrome • Spinal cord injuries

KEY POINTS

- Accelerated cardiometabolic disease is a serious health hazard after spinal cord injuries (SCI).
- Lifestyle intervention with diet and exercise remains the cornerstone of effective cardiometabolic syndrome (CMS) treatment.
- Behavioral approaches enhance compliance and benefits derived from both diet and exercise interventions and are necessary to assure that persons with SCI profit from intervention.
- Multitherapy strategies will likely be needed to control challenging component risks, such as gain in body mass, which has far reaching implications for maintenance of daily function as well as health.
- In cases where lifestyle approaches prove inadequate for risk management, pharmacologic control is now available through a population-tested monotherapy.
- Use of these clinical pathways will foster a more effective health-centered culture for stakeholders with SCI and their health care professionals.

CARDIOMETABOLIC RISKS IN SCI

Health hazards posed by all-cause cardiovascular disease (CVD) and co-morbid endocrine disorders are widely reported in persons with spinal cord injuries (SCI).[1–3] The contemporary descriptor cardiometabolic syndrome (CMS) represents a complex

Supported by grants from the National Institute for Disability and Rehabilitation Research #H133G080150, the Craig H. Neilsen Foundation #124683, and the Congressionally Mandated Medical Research Program - United States Department of Defense #W81XWH-10-1-1044 (SC090095).
[a] Department of Neurological Surgery, Miller School of Medicine, University of Miami, 1475 North West 12th Avenue, Miami, FL 33136, USA; [b] The Miami Project to Cure Paralysis, Miller School of Medicine, University of Miami, 1095 North West 14th Terrace, Lois Pope LIFE Center, Miami, FL 33136, USA; [c] Department of Rehabilitation Medicine, Miller School of Medicine, University of Miami, 1500 North West 12th Avenue, Suite 1409, Miami, FL 33136, USA
* Corresponding author.
E-mail address: mnash@med.miami.edu

Phys Med Rehabil Clin N Am 25 (2014) 573–604
http://dx.doi.org/10.1016/j.pmr.2014.04.006
1047-9651/14/$ – see front matter © 2014 Elsevier Inc. All rights reserved.

array of these hazards, which by evidence-based clinical diagnosis encompasses 5 component risks of central obesity, hypertriglyceridemia, low-plasma high-density lipoprotein cholesterol (HDL-C), hypertension, and fasting hyperglycemia (**Table 1**).[4–7] Left untreated, these risks promote atherosclerotic plaque formation and premature CVD, and when identified in clusters of 3 or more risks, confer the same clinical threat as frank diabetes or extant coronary artery disease.[6]

Special Concerns for Persons with SCI (Accelerated Risk and Specific Targets)

Convincing evidence supports the population-specific threat to persons with SCI for an accelerated trajectory of CMS, which is typically seen as component risks of central obesity,[8,9] impaired fasting glucose and frank diabetes,[10,11] dyslipidemia,[1,12] and (depending on the nature and level of injury) hypertension. Blood pressure, however, is a 2-sided issue in the SCI population. Persons with high-level SCI (T6 or above, where sympathetic nervous system control is likely compromised[13,14]) frequently suffer from hypotension.[15] Persons with lower-level injuries have similar hypertension issues as the general population.[16] Target levels for markers of these CMS risks have been established (see **Table 1**) for the general population but not specifically for SCI. In the absence of specific recommendations, general targets for lipid and glycemic markers may be adequate for persons with SCI. However, standard categories for common surrogate measures of obesity, such as waist circumference (WC) or body mass index (BMI), are not applicable for SCI and should be adjusted to greater than 94 cm WC[17] and $\geq$22 kg/m^2 BMI,[18] respectively.

THERAPEUTIC LIFESTYLE INTERVENTION

Guideline-driven interventions to reduce CMS risks follow a pathway that first eliminates drugs and biologic agents that might be causing the CMS, which would include tobacco use. Otherwise, little in the pharmacopeia of persons with SCI would cause or

Table 1
Cardiometabolic component risks

Risk	Criterion	
	ATP III	**WHO**
(Abdominal) obesity	• WC >40 inches (102 cm) for men • WC >35 inches (88 cm) for women • WC >37 inches (94 cm) for persons with SCI[a]	• WHR >0.90 for men • WHR >0.85 for women • BMI $\geq$30 kg/m^2 for men and women • BMI $\geq$22 kg/m^2 persons with SCI[a]
Triglycerides	• $\geq$150 mg/dL (1.7 mmol/L)	
HDL-cholesterol	• <40 mg/dL (1.03 mmol/L) for men • <50 mg/dL (1.29 mmol/L) for women	• <0.9 mmol/L for men • <1.0 mmol/L for women
Blood pressure	• $\geq$130/85 mm Hg, or use of medication for hypertension	• 160/90 mm Hg
Hyperglycemia	• FPG $\geq$100 mg/dL (5.6 mmol/L), or use of medication for hyperglycemia	• DM/IGT/IFG
Microalbuminuria	• N/A	• $\geq$20 µg/min, or albumin:creatinine ratio $\geq$20 mg/g

[a] Adjusted for SCI based on Refs.[17,18]

worsen the CMS. Thereafter, comprehensive therapeutic lifestyle intervention (TLI) focusing on changes of dietary, exercise, and behavioral components is instituted. If these measures fail to correct the hazard, pharmacotherapy becomes the default intervention. This article provides details for each of these risk countermeasures. A clinical pathway outlining the treatment decision-making in this respect is shown in **Fig. 1**.

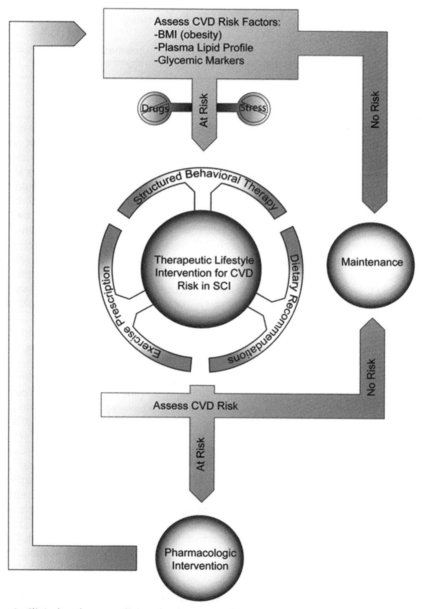

Fig. 1. Clinical pathway outlining the treatment decision-making for reducing cardiometabolic disease in SCI.

Dietary Component of TLI
Based on information from United States Department of Agriculture (USDA) Dietary Guidelines for Americans 2010,[19] adapted for SCI where applicable.

Key points

- Energy intake has to be balanced with output to avoid or reduce obesity and prevent or improve CVD risk.
- Diet recommendations for persons with SCI should follow general guidelines, including increasing whole grain, fruit, and vegetable intake, while reducing salt, simple sugar, saturated fat, and cholesterol intake.
- Specific evidence for persons with SCI is sparse and diet recommendations should follow general guidelines except for BMI targets and energy requirement estimates.

Diet Considerations—Energy Balance, Body Composition, and Malnutrition

Weight maintenance or weight loss is the primary goal of most diet interventions aimed at preventing and reducing obesity and CMS risk. Even modest amounts of body weight reduction can result in marked health benefits.[20,21] Energy (caloric) intake and output are the primary factors determining changes in weight and need to be balanced according to the desired goal (ie, if one desires weight loss one needs to achieve a negative balance [energy intake<energy output]). More specifically, body fat reduction while maintaining (or increasing) lean mass (ie, muscle) should be targeted in an effort to improve body composition. This goal is of particular relevance to the upper extremities in persons with SCI because upper extremity function is crucial for daily activities, pain, and independence.[22–24] Weight loss achieved by reducing caloric intake usually results in 14% to 24% loss in lean tissue mass[25,26] and should therefore be accompanied by an exercise regimen to avoid such losses[27] (see exercise section). In addition to energy balance, dietary interventions should also consider specific nutrition needs to avoid malnutrition (overconsumption and underconsumption of nutrients) and promote optimal health. These key concepts and considerations are explained in detail in discussion below and summarized in **Box 1**.

Assessing energy balance

To set caloric targets for weight loss or maintenance, current energy intake and output need to be assessed. The most direct way of assessing everyday energy intake is to measure all consumed foods and beverages and calculate caloric values from food labels. However, this may be cumbersome and time-consuming, particularly for persons with impaired hand function.[28,29] More practical may be the use of diet recall or food frequency questionnaires (preferably with instruction from a professional[30]) in combination with nutrition analysis software. Multiple different analysis software packages are available including a free online calculator from the USDA (SuperTracker[31]).

Energy output or total energy expenditure (TEE) comprises basal metabolic rate (BMR), physical activity (PA), and energy expenditure (EE) from the breakdown, digestion, absorption, and excretion of food (summed up as the thermic effect of food, TEF). Most TEE (>80%) is accounted for by the by BMR and PA (see exercise section).[32–34] Laboratory assessments of TEE are difficult and expensive and standard "field" techniques often overestimate TEE in persons with SCI.[34] Better estimates of TEE are achieved with specific questionnaires,[34] such as The Physical Activity Scale for Individuals with Physical Disabilities[35] or the Physical Activity Recall Assessment for People with Spinal Cord Injury.[36]

Box 1
Key concepts and considerations for dietary component of TLI

- Assess energy balance
  - Energy intake
    - Diet analysis
  - TEE
    - BMR/REE
    - PA/exercise
    - TEF
- Create caloric deficit
  - Reduce energy intake
    - Reduce calorie-dense foods
  - Increase EE
    - PA/exercise
    - TEF
- Malnutrition
  - Overconsumption of macronutrients
    - Fats, cholesterol, CHO
  - Underconsumption of micronutrients and fiber
    - Vitamin A, D, E, C, B5, and biotin
- Recommended diets
  - Mediterranean
  - DASH

Creating a caloric deficit

After assessing energy balance, a caloric deficit of 300 kcal or less should be created to elicit weight loss. Ideally, this should be from a combination of reduced caloric intake and increased expenditure, although the latter may be difficult for persons with SCI (see exercise section). To achieve the caloric deficit, people should reduce or eliminate primarily energy-dense food high in components associated with elevated CMS risk, such as saturated fats/trans fats, added/refined sugars, refined grains, and alcohol, as outlined in **Table 2**. Increased EE will largely depend on PA and body composition changes affecting BMR and may be difficult for persons with SCI (see exercise section). Increased TEF may contribute to a small extent. Little is known about specific foods that increase TEF, but generally TEF is higher for protein compared with other macronutrients (ie, carbohydrates and fats)[37,38] and may be positively affected by certain micronutrients (reviewed in Ref.[39]). The latter, however, mostly lacks rigorously controlled evidence[39] and should therefore be met with caution. Contrary to common belief, fiber does not seem to augment TEF[40–43] (unless it contains high amounts of polyphenols[44]) but may increase fecal energy loss.[45,46] Of note, people with SCI may have reduced TEF (12% of TEE vs 15% for able bodied [AB][33]). Although reduction of caloric intake is the key to weight loss, it should not decrease to less than 800 kcal/d and may have to be considerably higher depending on the individual's age, size, body composition, activity level, disease status, and other factors that affect

Table 2
Reduce or eliminate high caloric density foods

Food Component Associated with CVD Risk	Examples
Saturated fat (<7% of TEE)	Animal products (except fish), coconut/palm oil, pizza, pastries, tortillas, chips, fried foods, etc.
Trans fats	Margarines, snack foods, pre-prepared dessert, partially hydrogenated oils, etc.
Added sugars	Soda/sports/energy/fruit/tea drinks, cereals, candy, desserts, etc.
Refined grains	Breads, pizza, pastries, tortillas, chips, pasta, prepared foods (mixed dishes), crackers, cereals, etc.
Alcohol (≤1 drink for women, ≤2 for men)	Beer, wine, spirits, liquors, etc.

metabolism.[47–52] Reference values for age and gender have been published by the USDA but likely overestimate energy needs for persons with SCI because of their lower metabolically active mass and PA levels. Studies directly comparing resting energy expenditure (REE) between AB and persons with SCI report on average 10% lower energy requirements for adults with chronic SCI (although this difference is markedly reduced to only 1.4% when REE is normalized to body weight).[32,33,47,52] Average REE for adults with chronic SCI have been reported to range from 1392 to 1855 kcal/d for men[32,33,47,53–57] and 1042 to 1290 kcal/d for women.[32,53] These values likely better represent caloric needs of persons with SCI than those published for the general population and can be used as initial targets for caloric deficits.

Malnutrition

To maximize health benefits, diet interventions need to extend beyond mere caloric balance boundaries and ensure adequate nutrient intake to avoid deficiencies.[58] In addition, excess consumption of dietary components associated with CMS risk should be reduced or eliminated.[58] Dietary Reference Intakes (DRI) have been published by the USDA.[19] Generally, consumption of macronutrients is adequate or excessive for persons with SCI (particularly for fat and cholesterol intakes) with the exception of fiber.[19,28,30,59–64] Fiber is of particular concern for persons with SCI because their most common lipid abnormality is low HDL and fiber consumption is positively related to HDL levels.[65–68] However, high fiber intake (20–30 g/d) may stimulate undesirable changes in bowel function that differ from the non-disabled population, rendering high fiber diets impractical for persons with SCI.[69–71]

Because of the general eating habits of most Americans, several micronutrients are of concern because the likelihood of deficiency is high.[19] These nutrients include potassium, fiber, calcium, and vitamin D as well as iron and folate (women only).[19] Several other nutrients (**Table 3**) are of particular concern for persons with SCI because they are often underconsumed by this population (reviewed in Refs.[28,72]). In addition, sufficient consumption of biotin and vitamin B5 (pantothenic acid) may also be of concern to persons with SCI,[28] although DRIs have not been published by the USDA Dietary Guidelines.[19]

Correcting nutrient deficiencies/excess

If deficiencies are identified, the diet should be augmented with specific foods high in these nutrients. As mentioned above, macronutrient deficiency is rare (except for fiber) for persons with SCI, although sources of the nutrients need to be considered and

Table 3
Dietary reference intake of nutrients often underconsumed by persons with SCI based on USDA dietary guidelines

Nutrient, Unit	Women			Men		
	19–30 y	31–50 y	51+ y	19–30 y	31–50 y	51+ y
Vitamin A (RAE), mcg	700	700	700	900	900	900
Vitamin D,[a] mcg	15	15	15	15	15	15
Vitamin E (AT), mg	15	15	15	15	15	15
Vitamin C, mg	75	75	75	90	90	90
Biotin,[b] mcg	30	30	30	30	30	30
Vitamin B5,[b] mg	5	5	5	5	5	5

Abbreviations: AT, α-tocopherol; RAE, retinoic acid equivalents; TEI, total energy intake.
[a] Assuming minimal sun exposure.
[b] Values are not from USDA Dietary Guidelines but based on date from Yates et al,[145] 1998.

should be mainly from lean meats and seafood (protein), whole grains (carbohydrates), and unsaturated fatty acids (fats).[19] More likely deficiencies are in certain micronutrients (as indicated above). Foods containing nutrients of particular concern to SCI are listed in **Table 4**.[73–80]

Excess intake of macronutrients is common for persons with SCI[28] and should be reduced ideally through reduction of intake of those foods listed in **Table 2**. In addition, salt intake by persons with SCI generally exceeds recommended levels.[59–61,69] These levels are established for the general population because of the positive relation of salt intake with high blood pressure.[19] However, persons with SCI at T6 and above where sympathetic nervous system (SNS) control is likely compromised[13,14] frequently suffer from hypotension.[15] Therefore, increased salt intake particularly in the morning has been recommended for individuals suffering from hypotension.[81,82] In contrast, person with SCI but uncompromised SNS should reduce their salt intake in line with general guidelines (<2300 or 1500 mg/d based on age, ethnicity and disease status).[19]

Table 4
Foods containing micronutrients with reported deficiencies in SCI

Nutrient	Examples of Nutrient Containing Foods
Vitamin A	Liver, fish oil, broccoli, spinach, romaine, collard, turnip, mustard greens, squash, pumpkin, carrot, sweet potatoes, mango
Vitamin D[a]	Salmon, tuna, and mackerel (small amounts also in beef liver, cheese, egg yolks) Dietary supplement fact sheet: vitamin D
Vitamin E	Nuts, seeds, vegetable oils, spinach, romaine, collard, turnip, and mustard greens
Vitamin C	Citrus fruits, tomatoes, potatoes, red and green peppers, kiwifruit, broccoli, strawberries, brussel sprouts, and cantaloupe
Biotin	Brewer's yeast; cooked eggs, especially egg yolk; sardines; nuts (almonds, peanuts, pecans, walnuts) and nut butters; soybeans; other legumes (beans, black eyed peas); whole grains; cauliflower; bananas; and mushrooms
Vitamin B5	Meat, vegetables, cereal grains, legumes, eggs, and milk

[a] Sun exposure can yield a significant amount of Vitamin D.[146,147]

Recommended diets

Dietary recommendations for persons with SCI are usually in line with those adopted for the general population[19] with exceptions for energy intake and sodium targets, as outlined above. Two contemporary dietary strategies that have been proven to positively affect components of the CMS are Mediterranean-style diets and the dietary approaches to stop hypertension (DASH),[83,84] which are summarized in **Fig. 2**.

Exercise component of TLI

Based on (1) The World Health Organizations' Global Strategy on Diet, Physical Activity, and Health[85]; (2) The US Department of Health and Human Services Physical Activity Guidelines for Americans[86]; (3) The Exercise is Medicine's Health Care Providers' Action Guide[87]; and (4) SCI Action Canada.[88]

Key points

- Exercise absent caloric restriction is unlikely to induce weight loss.
- Exercise recommendations for adults with SCI to improve cardiometabolic risk factors are the same as for adults without disabilities.
- To improve health and wellness, persons with SCI should engage in at least 150 minutes of moderate intensity aerobic exercise each week, perform strength training exercises at least 2 times a week, and stretch at least 2 times a week.

Exercise Considerations—Role in Health and Weight Management

Exercise interventions should be applied with the primary objective of improving metabolic profiles and body composition (not mere weight loss per se). Nevertheless, exercise/PA interventions can augment caloric restriction to accelerate/maintain weight loss. However, as explained in discussion below, for most persons with SCI exercise as a monotherapy will be insufficient to induce weight loss. Although exercise interventions in isolation are unlikely to achieve weight loss for persons with SCI, they are effective for improving strength,[89,90] which in turn support daily independence. Strength gains are also typically associated with an underlying muscle gain and hence positive body composition changes. Over time, increased muscle mass could enhance resting metabolic rate and thus support TEE and weight management.

Exercise and Caloric Balance

Weight loss is achieved through a sustained negative caloric balance as described in the diet component above. Because of lower absolute peak aerobic levels,[91] reduced muscle mass available to expend calories,[92] and autonomic dysfunction[93] (above T6), persons with SCI burn 30% to 50% fewer calories than non-disabled persons during moderate to vigorous exercise intensities.[94] This decreased caloric capacity to burn calories requires increased exercise duration to achieve similar caloric expenditures. Given most non-disabled individuals are challenged to achieve the total weekly recommended PA amounts required to lose weight (60–90 min a day, 5 times a week), it is reasonable to assume the additional time required by persons with SCI (78–135 min a day, 5 times a week) to reach similar caloric expenditures will present an insurmountable obstacle for many. In addition, performing common modes of exercise for SCI such as pushing a wheelchair or using arm ergometry for extended periods of time may also increase the risk for shoulder and wrist overuse injury.

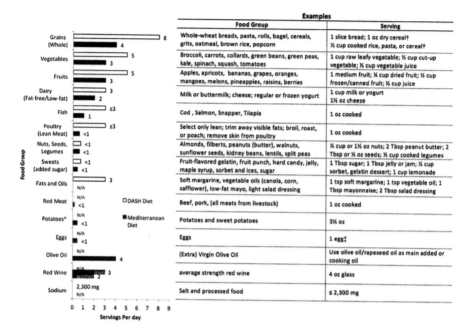

Fig. 2. Dietary recommendations based on the Mediterranean and DASH diets. *Note:* The Mediterranean-style diets are sometimes considered high in fat content and calories for sedentary populations, although the fats are generally monounsaturated and not the more atherogenic saturated fats. The DASH diet is usually prescribed for hypertension management to a greater degree than fat loss, although high intake of fruits and vegetables in the diet may favor the same weight reduction goals. ᵃ Potatoes and eggs are included in the vegetable and lean meat groups, respectively, for the DASH diet. ᵇ Serving sizes vary between $1/2$ cup and $1 1/4$ cups, depending on cereal type. Check the product's nutrition facts label. ᶜ Eggs are high in cholesterol; therefore, limit egg yolk intake to ≤ 4 per week. (*Data from* NIH National Heart, Lung and Blood Institute. Available at: http://www.nhlbi.nih.gov/health/health-topics/topics/dash/followdash.html; and Brooks G. Mediterranean diet: summary and chart. Available at: http://www.patient.co.uk/health/mediterranean-diet-summary-chart.)

PA Requirements for Weight Loss, Health, and Wellness

The PA levels required for weight loss are much greater than those required to support health and wellness gains (ie, improved cardiometabolic risk factors).[95] Nevertheless, the amount required to support health and wellness in persons with SCI is the same as required for the general population. The World Health Organization (WHO)[85] and the United States Department of Health and Human Services[86] state that guidelines for adults without disabilities can be valid for adults with disabilities. Both organizations note that adjustments can be made as needed to accommodate each individual's exercise capacity, health risks, or limitations. In as much as possible, people with SCI should be encouraged to achieve the minimum targets (**Table 5**).

Exercise Prescription

PA guidelines have been established to be easily comprehensible by the general population but implementation and adherence are greatly enhanced with health care provider guidance. When physician advice is coupled with an exercise plan, patients are 2 times more likely to exercise than those who receive advice but no exercise plan.[96] This increases to 3 times more likely to exercise when physician advice is coupled

Table 5
Target PA levels to improve health and wellness among persons with SCI

Aerobic PA			
Intensity[a]	Moderate		Vigorous

Weekly total[a]	≥150 min
	Can be accumulated in
	  bouts ≥10 min
	(eg, 30 min 5 d a wk)
	(eg, 15 min morning and
	  evening 5 d a wk)
		OR	≥75 min
			Can be accumulated in
			  bouts ≥10 min
			(eg, 15 min 5 d a wk)
			(eg, ~11 min every day of
			  the week)

Activity type	Any activity that achieves
	  the above
			Any activity that achieves
			  the above

Lay intensity guide[b]	"Somewhat hard," "you
	  can talk but not sing," or
	  is 5 or 6 on a 0 to 10 scale
			"Really hard," "you can't
			  say more than a few
			  words without pausing
			  for breath," or is 7 or 8 on
			  a 0 to 10 scale

AND	
Resistance training	
Frequency[a]	≥2 d per wk
Number of exercises	All major muscle groups[a] (~4–5 upper body exercises). (For shoulder health, be sure to include scapular stabilizer and posterior shoulder muscles.)
Sets and repetitions[a]	3 sets of 8–12 repetitions (each exercise)
Weight[b]	Enough to create a feeling of "quite challenged" at the end of each set

AND	
Upper extremity stretching	
Frequency[c]	2–3 d per wk
Areas to stretch[c]	Chest and anterior shoulders & perform full range of motion for all upper extremity joints
When stretching[c]	Apply a gentle, prolonged stretch to each area of tightness

[a] WHO PA recommendation for adults ages 18–64.
[b] Lay Intensity Guide from SCIAction Canada.
[c] Stretching guideline from Consortium for Spinal Cord Medicine's Upper Extremity Preservation Guideline.

with an exercise plan and regular follow-up queries.[96] Persons with SCI indicate a preference for obtaining PA information from their health care provider.[97] Thus, there is a strong potential that SCI health care providers can increase the PA level of their patients by providing exercise prescriptions.

A Health Care Providers Action Guide from the Exercise is Medicine (EIM) initiative is available online.[87] This initiative is a joint effort by the American College of Sports Medicine (ACSM) and the American Medical Association "to make physical activity and exercise a standard part of a global disease prevention and medical treatment." It is widely supported by professional societies, including the American Academy of Physical Medicine and Rehabilitation (AAPMR), American Physical Therapy Association, American Heart Association (AHA), and the American Osteopathic Association. The Health Care Providers guide is available on the EIM Web site. The guide contains a 4-step PA prescription process, which should be adjusted for SCI as outlined in **Box 2**.

Box 2
Recommended adjustments for patient with SCI to EIM Health Care Providers Action Guide Four-Step Physical Activity Prescription Process

Step

1. If patient is not currently exercising and unwilling to start an exercise program, advise of risks of inactivity (eg, loss of independence, weight gain) and encourage them to exercise.

   i. Recent SCI-specific research indicates loss-framed messages (eg, inactivity risks) result in greater increases in PA than gain-framed messages (eg, PA benefits).[148]

2. Administer Physical Activity Readiness Questionnaire Plus (PAR-Q+), which includes SCI-specific clearance questions/concerns.

3. No SCI-specific adaptation necessary.

4. In addition to aerobic and strength training, recommend a stretching component to help protect the shoulders from overuse. **Table 5** presents all components of an exercise prescription.

Specific Considerations for SCI

A "complete" exercise prescription includes aerobic and strength training. In addition, regular flexibility exercise (ie, stretching) should be encouraged to help protect the shoulders from overuse. **Table 5** presents all components of an exercise prescription.

Aerobic exercise considerations
To support health and wellness, the WHO recommends adults aged 18 to 65 perform at least 150 minutes of moderate intensity or 75 minutes of vigorous aerobic PA each week,[85] translating to 30 minutes of moderate intensity or 15 minutes of vigorous intensity activity 5 days a week. Aerobic activity can be accumulated in bouts as short as 10 minutes. For a person with SCI, moderate intensity is described as "somewhat hard," "you can talk but not sing," or is 5 or 6 on a 0 to 10 scale.[88] Vigorous intensity is described as "really hard," "you can't say more than a few words without pausing for breath," or is 7 or 8 on a 0 to 10 scale.[88]

Muscle strengthening considerations
In addition, WHO recommends muscle strengthening activities involving major muscle groups be done 2 or more days a week. For persons with SCI, the specific recommendation is at least 3 sets of 8 to 12 repetitions for each major muscle group 2 times a week.[88] The weight should be enough to create a feeling of "quite challenged" at the end of each set. For most persons with SCI, 4 to 5 different upper extremity exercises should be sufficient to address all upper extremity muscles. It is very important to ensure scapular stabilizers and posterior shoulder muscles are strengthened to protect the shoulder against overuse injuries.

Stretching considerations
In conjunction with strengthening the scapular stabilizers and posterior shoulder muscles, it is critical that persons with SCI stretch their chest (pectoralis muscles) and anterior shoulders (long head of the biceps). The Clinical Practice Guidelines recommend that persons with SCI should stretch 2 to 3 times a week. During each stretching session, they should apply a gentle, prolonged stretch to each area of tightness in the neck, upper trunk, and each arm.[98] In addition, during each stretching session they should perform full range-of-motion exercises for all upper extremity joints.[98]

Referral to a Clinical Exercise Professional

In lieu of or in conjunction with writing an exercise prescription, a health care provider can refer their patient to a clinical exercise professional. Examples of clinical exercise professionals include ACSM-certified clinical exercise specialists and ACSM-registered exercise physiologists. The EIM initiative suggests health care professionals develop a local network of clinical exercise professionals to whom they can refer their patients. By developing a local network, health care providers can ensure local clinical exercise professionals are well versed in the needs, limitations, and health risks of persons with SCI. Alternatively, a local clinical exercise professional can be found by searching the ACSM ProFinder information database.[99]

Managing Shoulder Pain

Upper limb injury is a serious concern for persons undertaking upper extremity exercise, as the prevalence of shoulder pain and injury is 30% to 60% after SCI.[100,101] If shoulder pain is present, circuit training[24] and anterior stretching/posterior strengthening regimens[102,103] are effective treatment options. The exercise prescription can be tailored as needed to minimize pain and injury until more intense exercise is tolerated. This approach is consistent with recommendations for comprehensive upper limb preservation from the Consortium for Spinal Cord Medicine.[98]

Behavioral component of TLI
Adapted from the joint American College of Cardiology (ACC)/AHA task force[19,104] and intended to reflect the behavior modification therapy of the Diabetes Prevention Program (DPP).[105] Modified for SCI where applicable.

Key points

- A comprehensive TLI for CMS risk includes structured behavior modification therapy.
- Key behavioral outcome objectives include
  1. *Education/instruction* on diet and exercise components and role in lowering CVD risk
  2. *Self-monitoring* of body weight, caloric intake, and PA levels, and
  3. Understanding psychosocial barriers and developing *cognitive strategies* to overcome barriers to diet and exercise goals.

Behavioral Modification

Evidence of current CMS prevention guidelines has been set forth by the ACC/AHA and consists of a collective series of documents outlining the assessment, treatment, and management of CMS risk factors, with particular attention to blood cholesterol, overweight, and obesity. Specifically, within the content of the overweight and obesity guidelines, it states that one of the principle components of an *"effective high-intensity...lifestyle intervention"* is the *"use of behavioral strategies to facilitate adherence"* to weight management recommendations. It is asserted that this therapy should provide a *"structured behavioral change program."* As a part of a comprehensive TLI, comprised of diet, PA, and behavior therapy, there is a *"high-to-moderate"* strength of evidence (derived from randomized control trials, meta-analysis, and quality observational studies) for efficacy in facilitating weight loss, when compared with *"usual," "minimal"* care, or no-treatment in the short term (6 months), intermediate (6–12 months), or long term (>1 year).

Key aspects

Several behavioral intervention aspects influence the overall effectiveness of a comprehensive TLI and include frequency and duration of treatment, individual versus group sessions, and onsite versus telephone/e-mail contact. The key behavioral outcome objectives summarized by the ACC/AHA are also outlined extensively in the landmark DPP behavioral program and include: (a) instruction on components of weight management (diet and exercise) and role in lowering CVD risk factors; (b) continuous *"self-monitoring"* with respect to body weight, food intake and composition, and PA level; and (c) cognitive restructuring and developing strategies to overcome psychosocial barriers to program compliance. Data from the DPP report both significant weight loss and a 58% decrease in the incidence of type 2 diabetes mellitus[106] following a structured TLI, consisting of nutrition, exercise, and behavioral weight management. Importantly, the DPP target, greater than or equal to 7% weight loss, was successful in maintaining low-diabetes-rate onset, as reported in a separately designed DPP outcome study (median follow-up of 5.7 years),[107] demonstrating effective long-term lifestyle change and cardiometabolic health benefit.

Several major CVD risk factors,[12,108–116] including overweight/obesity,[59,117–119] are established as pervasive in chronic SCI. Research outlining the impaired psychosocial health, quality of life, and subjective well-being following SCI is extensive (reviewed in Ref.[120]) and, correspondingly, emerging research supports the effectiveness of cognitive behavioral therapy (reviewed in Ref.[121]) in improving health-related quality of life and psychological issues. Although the scope of behavior therapy reviewed was in relation to depression, anxiety, coping, and adjustment post-SCI, it illustrates the potential effectiveness of directed behavior change on secondary complications in SCI.

Recent developments

More recent reports, including the authors' group, have focused on barriers to exercise participation[122,123] and factors influencing dietary status and nutritional habits,[28,29] addressing physical and environmental challenges, and inadequacies in education and psychosocial support, as relevant contributors to these imprudent lifestyle choices, which promote CVD and overweight/obesity risk. As such, a directed cognitive behavioral program as a component of management guidelines for a comprehensive population-specific lifestyle intervention is greatly in need. To our knowledge, there has been one recent uncontrolled study[124] administering dietary and exercise *"advice"* given in 3 *"behavioral change"* consultations over 3 months, and reporting weight loss and reduced BMI. Still, there remain no comprehensive reports of directed intervention trials for obesity and CMS risk factors in SCI. Currently underway, our group is conducting a TLI trial for cardiometabolic disease prevention/treatment in the SCI population. The TLI integrates dietary recommendations, exercise prescription, and structured behavioral therapy, consisting of a 16-session educational program modified from DPP principles to address the specific needs of persons with SCI (**Table 6**). Preliminary data confirm the effectiveness of the TLI in significantly reducing major CVD risk factors, including body weight, BMI, plasma lipid profile, and glycemic markers. These results highlight the potential effectiveness of a TLI for cardiometabolic disease in SCI.

PHARMACOTHERAPEUTIC APPROACHES

Lifestyle intervention incorporating caloric restriction, nutrient modification, and increased daily caloric expenditure usually serve as effective first-line treatments for CMS risks. However, loss of body fat may require unrealistic caloric restriction, and basal and exercise-induced caloric expenditures are decreased in patients with

Table 6
Strategic behavioral modification therapy

	Session	Topic	SCI Considerations	Example of Specific Advice/Information
Diet and exercise principles and goals	1	• Introduction to TLI • Explanation of goals	• Emphasize accelerated CVD risk • Independence	• Physical deconditioning and immobility lead to reduced caloric requirement → Greater likelihood for excess caloric intake • Enhance strength/lose weight to facilitate transfers
	2	• Focus on self-monitoring • Body weight/BMI • Diet (Intake) • Exercise (expenditure)	• At risk BMI ≥22 m/kg^2 • At risk WC 94 cm	• Measure body weight weekly • Take daily food log • Take daily exercise log
	3	• Emphasis on healthy eating • Understanding food labels • Discuss healthy food alternatives	• Limitations to accessing foods • Strategies to make healthier food choices accessible • Discuss specific nutritional deficiencies	• Discuss difficulties getting to and/or shopping at supermarket • Have fruits and vegetables in reach at home • Whole grains vs refined/processed carbs • Vitamins A, D, E, C, B5, biotin, fiber
	4	• Discuss ways to reduce fat intake	• Does caregiver/aide understand healthier food choices	• Discuss calorie dense foods, fat grams • Explain difference/sources of saturated vs unsaturated fats
	5	• Introduction to PA principles in weight control and CMS	• Understanding physiologic limitations in response to exercise • Discuss functional benefit	• Discuss variable responses to exercise (consider level of injury) • Activities of daily living—weight/strength and wheelchair transfer
	6	• Tailoring PA options for maintenance beyond TLI	• Discussing appropriate/feasible aerobic and anaerobic activities • Exploring facilities that provide adaptive support	• Wheelchair sports • In-home exercise (Therabands, Exergaming)[127]
	7	• Discuss principles of energy balance between calories and PA • Discuss principles of health maintenance from exercise	• Discuss how activities of daily living are unique in terms of EE	• Pushing a wheelchair burns less calories than walking a similar distance • Discuss risk of overuse injuries

8	Introduce principles of stimulus control • In preventing unhealthy eating • In maintain PA goals	• Difficulties preparing healthier foods • Absence of convenient activities/facilities for disability	• Do not have unhealthy foods in visible areas • Do not eat while involved in other recreation (ie, watching TV) • Get schedules of classes that are available so that you can plan ahead
Psychosocial issues and strategies			
9	• Present 5-step model of problem solving 1. Define problem in detail 2. Brainstorm options 3. Pick an option to try 4. Make positive action plan 5. Try it and assess	• Preparing healthy foods independently • Access to public activity facilities	• Discuss specific problems that may be inherent to the disability and brainstorm action plans that are appropriate
10	• Introduce principles of eating/exercising away from home • Planning ahead • Assertion • Stimulus control • Healthy food choices	• Identifying healthy restaurants and exercise facilities that are adaptive to disability	• If the choice is available, look up and suggest healthier places to eat • It is important to be vocal as to your needs to both restaurant employees and those in your social network
11	• Identifying negative thoughts • "All or nothing" • Excuse • "Should" • "Not as good as" • Give up • Coping strategies • Catch yourself • Stop yourself • Replace with positive thought	• Prevalence of depression	• It is common to compare health-related outcomes to others, either disabled or not, rather than focus on individual progress (ie, a "not as good as" thought)
12	• Discuss the concept of slips • As a natural part of lifestyle change • Tips to recover behavior modification	• Individuals experience inherent health complications • Need planning/strategies to cope	• Discuss infection, sores, AD that may interfere with diet/exercise consistency

(continued on next page)

Table 6
(continued)

Session	Topic	SCI Considerations	Example of Specific Advice/Information

13	• Discuss boredom in TLI program
	  • Dietary
	  • Activity—F.I.T.T.
		• Exercise intensity (as HR)
		• Central vs peripheral RPE
			• For low-level paraplegia, may more closely reflect guidelines than higher-level paraplegia and tetraplegia
			• Central is a more appropriate surrogate for intensity in upper level injury

14	• Discuss strategies for managing social cues
	  • Stressful (negative)
	  • Supportive (positive)
		• Vocalize study and health needs and goals to support group to change the landscape of social environment	• Friends/family members providing energy-dense "comfort" food during rehabilitation and beyond may be counterproductive

15	• Summary of stress management principles
	  • Define/identify stressors
	  • Explore individual signs of stress
	  • Strategies to manage unavoidable stress
	  • Strategies to prevent additional stress
		• Secondary health concerns (AMS risk) are a constant stressor	• Reiterate that intervention represents a modified lifestyle that must be maintained

16	• Focus on enhancing motivation	• Independence (activities of daily living)	• Set specific activity goals (ie, wheel-chair transfer) • Using a manual rather than powered wheelchair

Abbreviation: F.I.T.T., frequency intensity time type.

tetraplegia because of diminished active muscle mass and adrenergic dysfunction accompanying injury above the level of spinal sympathetic outflow. In addition, persons with SCI have limited capacity to burn fat during exercise.[125–128] When first-line approaches of diet and exercise fail to modify risk, evidence-based guidelines and current practice standards recommend pharmacotherapy. Very little evidence exists regarding pharmacotherapy for CMS specific to persons with SCI. Approaches developed and tested in the general population serve as general guides, representing default guidelines until SCI-specific evidence is available.

Drug Approaches to Treat Obesity

Three prescription drugs are currently FDA approved for weight loss, although none have been studied in a randomized controlled trial examining persons with SCI. **Table 7** identifies "on-label" drugs for weight loss, approved uses, drug mechanisms, common adverse effects, and "off-label" drugs for weight loss marketed as appetite suppressants ("anorexigenics").

Drug Approaches to Treat Hyperglycemia

The American Diabetes Association (ADA) defines hyperglycemia in nonpregnant adults as glycated hemoglobin (HbA_{1c}) greater than or equal to 6.5% (performed in a laboratory using an National Glycohemoglobin Standardization Program (NGSP)-certified method standardized to the DCCT assay and in the absence of unequivocal hyperglycemia results to be confirmed by repeat testing); or fasting plasma glucose (fasting defined as no caloric intake for 8 hours or more) greater than or equal to 126 mg/dL (7.0 mmol/L); or 2-hour plasma glucose greater than or equal to 200 mg/dL (11.1 mmol/L) during an OGTT (75 g)[2]; or random plasma glucose greater than or equal to 200 mg/dL (11.1 mmol/L) (in persons with symptoms of hyperglycemia or hyperglycemic crisis).[129]

Current ADA treatment recommendations for hyperglycemia[130] are shown in **Box 3**, whereas candidate drugs to treat hyperglycemia after SCI have been reviewed by Goldberg.[131] Eleven classes of oral medication are currently approved to treat hyperglycemia in people with type 2 diabetes. Most of these agents lower HbA_{1c} levels by 0.5% to 2.0%. Depending on pretreatment HbA_{1c} levels, effective treatment may require more than one agent. Recent evidence-based guidelines, including a consensus algorithm for initiation and adjustment of therapy, identified metformin as a preferred first-line agent,[132] as it is less prone to cause hypoglycemia and water retention than other agents, may promote minor weight loss, and is available in generic formulation. Recommended add-ons to achieve A1c targets are glucagon-like peptide-1 receptor agonists (Byetta and Victoza). None of these agents has been systematically tested in persons with SCI, although no available evidence suggests that either benefits or adverse effects would differ from those reported. To the authors' knowledge, no specific data on persons with SCI are currently available; however, preliminary evidence from our laboratory suggests potential benefits of salsalate monotherapy on fasting and postprandial plasma glucose.[133]

Drug Approaches to Treat Dyslipidemia

Five classes of agents are currently used to treat lipid disorders occurring in the general population (**Table 8**). Goldberg has previously described suggested drug choices and nuances for medication selection in persons with SCI.[131] Until recently, need for intervention on an atherogenic lipid profile was determined by the National Cholesterol Education Program Adult Treatment Panel (ATP) III guidelines,[134] which based treatment on whether low-density lipoprotein (LDL) measured in fasting blood plasma

Table 7
Prescription drugs approved for obesity treatment

Drug	Synonyms and Approvals	Drug Description/Comments	Common Adverse Effects
Orlistat	Sold as Xenical (Rx) and Alli (OTC). Xenical: adults and children ages 12 and older; Alli: adults only 2 y as an adjunct to diet and exercise	A gastrointestinal lipase inhibitor that acts by inhibiting the absorption of dietary fats No evidence suggests that use is suitable in patients with a neurogenic bowel	Stomach pain, gas, diarrhea, and leakage of oily stools Note: Rare cases of hepatotoxicity reported; should not be taken with cyclosporine
Lorcaserin	Sold as Belviq for adult use	Decreases food consumption and promotes satiety by selectively activating 5-HT$_{2C}$ receptors on hypothalamic anorexigenic proopiomelano-cortin neurons	Headaches, dizziness, fatigue, nausea, dry mouth, cough, and constipation. Should not be taken with selective serotonin reuptake inhibitors and monoamine oxidase inhibitor medications WARNINGS for serotonin syndrome or neuroleptic malignant syndrome–like reactions
Phentermine-topiramate	Sold as Qsymia for adult use	Phentermine is a sympathomimetic amine with anorexigenic properties Topiramate is an anticonvulsant promoting appetite suppression and satiety enhancement	Fatigue, paresthesias of hands and feet, dizziness, dysgeusia (particularly with carbonated beverages), insomnia, constipation, and dry mouth MAY LEAD TO BIRTH DEFECTS. DO NOT TAKE IF PREGNANCY MAY OCCUR.
Other appetite suppressants	("off-label" for weight loss): ■ Phentermine ■ Benzphetamine ■ Diethylpropion ■ Phendimetrazine (and other names) Adults (Note: FDA approved up to 12 wk)	Generally classified as sympathomimetic amines and administered as anorectic drugs (schedule IV controlled substances)	Xerostomia, restlessness, nervousness, euphoria, agitation, arrhythmia, tachycardia, hypertension, diarrhea, vomiting, headache, rash, urinary frequency, facial edema, unpleasant taste, urticaria, impotence, changes in libido

---

Box 3
ADA 2013 Guidelines for type 2 diabetes treatment: hyperglycemia

- Metformin
  - Preferred initial therapy (if tolerated and not contraindicated)
- Consider insulin therapy
  - With or without other agents at outset in newly diagnosed patients with markedly symptomatic and/or elevated blood glucose levels or A1C
- Add second oral agent, GLP-1 receptor agonist, or insulin
  - If noninsulin monotherapy at maximal tolerated dose does not achieve or maintain A1C target over 3–6 months
- Choice of pharmacologic therapy should be based on a patient-centered approach
- Consider
  - Efficacy
  - Cost
  - Potential side effects
  - Effects on weight
  - Comorbidities
  - Hypoglycemia risk
  - Patient preferences
- Insulin therapy is eventually needed for many patients due to progressive nature of type 2 diabetes

---

exceeded a criterion target computed from an array of CVD risk factors and prediction equations. Dyson-Hudson and Nash have reviewed testing methods and systematic approaches to ATP III–based treatment decision-making.[135] In general, an intermediate CVD risk stratification was used to define need for treatment, which included

Table 8
Candidate drugs for treating dyslipidemia and expected effects on key elements of the lipid profile

Drug Class	Candidate Drugs	TG %Δ	LDL-C %Δ	HDL-C %Δ
HMG-CoA reductase inhibitors: "Statins"	• Atorvastatin (Lipitor) • Lovastatin (Mevacor) • Pravastatin (Pravacol) • Rasuvastatin (Crestor) • Simvastatin (Zocor)	↓ 10–30	↓ 25–55	↑ 5–15
Cholesterol uptake blocker	• Ezitamibe (Zetia)	↓ 5–15	↓ 15–20	N/A
Bile-acid sequestrates	• Cholestyramine (Questran) • Colesevelam (Welchol) • Colestipol (Colestid)	↑↓ 10–20	↑↓ 20–20	N/A
Niacin releaser	• Niaspan	↓ 10–30	↓ 5–25	↑ 10–35
Fibric acid derivatives	• Atromid (Clofibrate) • Tricor (Fenofibrate) • Lopid (Gemfibrozil)	↓ 30–50	↓ 0–5	↑ 5–20

individuals having Framingham scores of 10% to 20% in the 10-year event risk category, and whose LDL-C levels are greater than 130 mg/dL, or greater than 100 mg/dL in the presence of risk factors including age, hypertension, and/or cigarette smoking or high-sensitivity C-reactive protein greater than 3 μg/L.

More recent guidelines focusing less on lipoprotein targets and more on population risk and need for intervention have been jointly recommended by the AHA and ACC.[136] This change is based on landmark studies showing that improvements in lipoprotein targets do not necessarily lead to better disease outcomes or lower event rates. The guidelines also identify HMG-CoA reductase inhibitors (syn: "statins") as the drug family of choice to anchor both primary and secondary interventions, as they are the most widely studied and have established benefits on disease endpoints and event rates. The guidelines designate 4 different groups for primary and secondary intervention:

1. Individuals who have already had an event and who have CVD (ie, myocardial infarction, unstable angina, stroke, or peripheral vascular disease) become "secondary prevention patients" and are considered at highest risk. They are placed on a high-dose statin (**Table 9**). Measurement of their lipids is not needed, as it is known that prescribing the maximum dose of a statin will maximally reduce their risk for having another event.
2. Individuals with LDL cholesterol level greater than or equal to 190 mg/dL are also considered to be at "very high risk" and are treated with intensive dose statin therapy.
3. Individuals aged 40 to 75 years with diabetes (regardless of type) are considered to be at high risk and are placed on statin therapy. Dosing as moderate intensity or high intensity is based on whether their 10-year risk for an event is greater than or equal to 7.5%. However, they are all put on a statin if they are between the ages of 40 and 75 years.
4. All individuals aged 40 to 75 years who fit within a pooled risk equation identifying a 10-year risk for a CVD event, where statin treatment is indicated if the risk is greater than or equal to 7.5%.

A clinical pathway for treatment decision-making is shown in **Fig. 3**.

Table 9
High-intensity, moderate-intensity, and low-intensity statin therapy (used in the RCTs reviewed by the expert panel)

Intensity	Drug Dose	Effects
Low	Simvastatin 10 mg Pravastatin 10–20 mg Lovastatin 20 mg Fluvastatin 20–40 mg Pitavastatin 1 mg	Daily dose lowers LDL-C on average, by <30%
Medium	Atorvastatin 10 (20) mg Rosuvastatin (5) 10 mg Simvastatin 20–40 mg Pravastatin 40 (80) mg Lovastatin 40 mg Fluvastatin XL 80 mg Fluvastatin 40 mg bid Pitavastatin 2–4 mg	Daily dose lowers LDL-C on average, by approximately 30% to <50%
High	Atorvastatin (40–80 mg) Rosuvastatin 29 (40) mg	Daily dose lowers LDL-C on average by approximately ≥50%

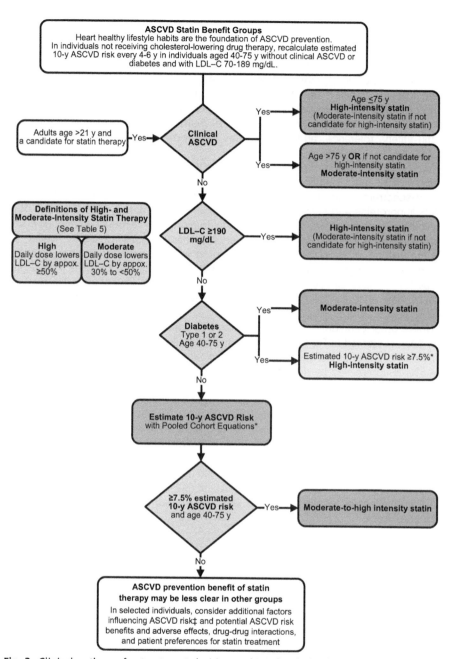

Fig. 3. Clinical pathway for treatment decision-making for dyslipidemia. *, Percent reduction in LDL–C can be used as an indication of response and adherence to therapy, but is not in itself a treatment goal; †, The Pooled Cohort Equations can be used to estimate 10-year ASCVD risk in individuals with and without diabetes. A downloadable spreadsheet enabling estimation of 10-year and lifetime risk for ASCVD and a web-based calculator are available at http://my.americanheart.org/cvriskcalculator and http://www.cardiosource. org/science-and-quality/practice-guidelines-and-quality-standards/2013-prevention-guideline-tools.aspx. (*From* Stone NJ, Robinson J, Lichtenstein AH, et al. 2013 ACC/AHA guideline on the treatment of blood cholesterol to reduce atherosclerotic cardiovascular risk in adults a report of the American College of Cardiology/American Heart Association task force on practice guidelines. J Am Coll Cardiol 2013; p.15; with permission.)

Unfortunately, the recent recommendations may have questionable application to persons with SCI, as (1) statins are not the best drugs for correcting the most prominent lipid abnormality after SCI (ie, low HDL-C)[137]; (2) statin-induced myositis[138] may challenge upper extremity function in persons who must use their arms for most daily activities, including wheelchair propulsion; and (3) a clinical trial testing statin safety, tolerance, and effectiveness has never been conducted on persons with SCI.

Nicotinic acid (Niacin) in extended release (ER) formulation represents a tested alternative to use of statins in persons with SCI. Niacin is an older, inexpensive broad-spectrum drug that decreases concentrations of all atherogenic plasma lipids/lipoproteins and is the most effective agent for increasing HDL-C levels.[139] In crystalline (ie, intermediate-release) form, the drug provokes a robust cutaneous flushing, thus compromising patient tolerance when therapeutically dosed. However, an ER formulation of niacin (Niaspan) administered with a prostaglandin antagonist (ie, 325 mg ASA) and gradual dose escalation reduces this discomfort.[140] The therapeutic response to Niacin directly addresses the CMS component risk of low HDL and addresses low HDL as the most common lipid disorder sustained by persons with SCI.[141]

Unlike other candidate drugs for treating SCI-associated dyslipidemia, niacin ER has been subjected to RCT in persons with SCI.[142] Results of 48 weeks of treatment on a dose-escalation schedule showed significant increases in fasting HDL-C levels (24.5%) accompanied by dose-dependent lowering of total cholesterol (TC) and TG (**Fig. 4**) decreases in the global risk predictor ratios of TC/HDL and LDL/HDL, LDL levels, and TC levels. No evidence of sustained hepatotoxicity or hyperglycemia was observed. Treatment-emergent withdrawals (12.9%) accompanied flushing (n = 1), hypotension/presyncope (n = 1), and diarrhea (n = 2), although event rates were lower than those reported for the same agent when treating non-disabled individuals. Although ER niacin use requires diligence in dose escalation, pretreatment with aspirin to suppress the accompanying flush, and abstention from spicy foods, alcohol, and hot showers in the pretreatment period, its use as a monotherapy is safe, tolerated, and effective for most persons with chronic tetraplegia, and it is expected, also paraplegia.

Drug Approaches to Treat Hypertension

Pharmacotherapeutic approaches to hypertension management in the United States have been defined by various sources including the Seventh Report of the Joint

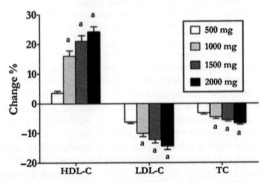

Fig. 4. Results of 48 weeks of Niaspan treatment on a dose-escalation schedule in fasting HDL-C, LDL-C, and TC levels. [a] Significant difference (P<.05).

Table 10
Hypertension treatment recommendations and blood pressure targets

Sponsor (Year)	Patient Assessment	Target BP (mm Hg)	Initial Drug Choices
JNC 7 (2003)	Stage 1 hypertension (SBP 140–159 or DBP 90–99)	<140/90	Thiazide diuretic (for most patients), ACE inhibitor, ARB, β-blocker, CCB, or combination
	Stage 2 hypertension (SBP ≥160 or DBP ≥100)	<140/90	Two-drug combination for most patients (thiazide diuretics plus ACE inhibitor, ARB, β-blocker, or CCB)
	Compelling disease indication	<130/80	1st: ACE inhibitor or ARB 2nd: thiazide diuretic 3rd: β-blocker, or CCB
AHA and ACC (2007 & 2008)	Primary prevention	<130/80	1st: ACE inhibitor or ARB
	Framingham risk score <10%	<140/90	ACE inhibitor or ARB, CCB, thiazide diuretic, or combination in needed
	Framingham risk score ≥10%	<130/80	ACE inhibitor (or ARB), CCB, thiazide diuretic, or combination if needed
High CAD risk	Diabetes mellitus	<130/80	1st: ACE inhibitor or ARB 2nd: thiazide diuretic 3rd: β-blocker, or CCB
	Chronic kidney disease	<130/80	1st: ACE inhibitor or ARB
CAD	Chronic stable angina Unstable angina Prior acute MI (NSTEMI or STEMI)	<130/80	1st: β-blocker, ACE inhibitor, or ARB 2nd: thiazide diuretic 3rd: CCB
	CAD risk equivalent, carotid artery disease (prior stroke or TIA)	<130/80	1st: ACE inhibitor (or ARB) or thiazide diuretic 2nd: CCB

Abbreviations: ACE, angiotensin converting enzyme inhibitor; ARB, angiotensin-2 receptor blocker; BP, blood pressure; CAD, coronary artery disease; CCB, calcium channel blocker; DBP, diastolic blood pressure; SBP, systolic blood pressure.

National Committee on Prevention, Detection, Evaluation, and Treatment of High Blood Pressure,[143] and joint statements from the AHA and American Society of Hypertension (summarized in Ref.[143]). More recent guidelines diverge from earlier recommendations that set grounded hypertension treatment at pressures greater than 140/90 mm Hg. Differences remain between the guideline recommendations with respect to selected pressure targets and first-line drug choices, although common elements include more conservative blood pressure targets (130/80 mm Hg) and drug therapy for primary prevention of hypertension in patients with elevated Framingham risk score. These same targets apply to patients with symptomatic coronary disease, and compelling conditions including diabetes and other comorbidities. Population-specific targets and recommended drugs therapies are shown in **Table 10**.[144] None of these agents have been systematically tested in persons with SCI, although no available evidence suggests that benefits or adverse effects would differ from those currently reported. As mentioned above, any treatment of hypertension needs to be evaluated in light of the nature and level of injury.

SUMMARY

A disconcerting number of people with SCI develop component risks for CMS as they age with their disability. These risks coalesce to comprise a frank diagnosis of the disorder in an alarming number of these individuals. Evaluation and diagnosis of the CMS now fall within the framework of an evidence-based clinical pathway that systematically assesses risk and defines uniform approaches to both individual risk containment and overall disease management.

REFERENCES

1. Nash MS, Mendez AJ. A guideline-driven assessment of need for cardiovascular disease risk intervention in persons with chronic paraplegia. Arch Phys Med Rehabil 2007;88(6):751–7.
2. Groah SL, Nash MS, Ward EA, et al. Cardiometabolic risk in community-dwelling persons with chronic spinal cord injury. J Cardiopulm Rehabil Prev 2011;31(2):73–80.
3. Bauman WA, Spungen A. Endocrinology and metabolism after spinal cord injury. Spinal cord medicine. Philadelphia: Lippincott Williams & Wilkins; 2002. p. 164–80.
4. Ford ES. Prevalence of the metabolic syndrome defined by the International Diabetes Federation among adults in the US. Diabetes Care 2005;28(11):2745–9.
5. Alberti KG, Zimmet PZ. Definition, diagnosis and classification of diabetes mellitus and its complications. Part 1: diagnosis and classification of diabetes mellitus provisional report of a WHO consultation. Diabet Med 1998;15(7):539–53.
6. Ford ES. Risks for all-cause mortality, cardiovascular disease, and diabetes associated with the metabolic syndrome: a summary of the evidence. Diabetes Care 2005;28(7):1769–78.
7. Expert Panel on Detection, Evaluation, and Treatment of High Blood Cholesterol in Adults. Executive summary of the third report of the national cholesterol education program (ncep) expert panel on detection, evaluation, and treatment of high blood cholesterol in adults (Adult Treatment Panel III). JAMA 2001;285(19):2486–97.
8. Gorgey AS, Gater DR. Prevalence of obesity after spinal cord injury. Top Spinal Cord Inj Rehabil 2007;12(4):1–7.

9. Gater DR. Obesity after spinal cord injury. Phys Med Rehabil Clin N Am 2007; 18(2):333–51.

10. Duckworth WC, Solomon SS, Jallepalli P, et al. Glucose intolerance due to insulin resistance in patients with spinal cord injuries. Diabetes 1980;29(11):906–10.

11. Bauman WA, Spungen AM. Coronary heart disease in individuals with spinal cord injury: assessment of risk factors. Spinal Cord 2008;46(7):466–76.

12. Bauman W, Spungen A, Zhong Y, et al. Depressed serum high density lipoprotein cholesterol levels in veterans with spinal cord injury. Spinal Cord 1992; 30(10):697–703.

13. Alan N, Ramer LM, Inskip JA, et al. Recurrent autonomic dysreflexia exacerbates vascular dysfunction after spinal cord injury. Spine J 2010;10(12):1108–17.

14. Cragg J, Krassioukov A. Autonomic dysreflexia. CMAJ 2012;184(1):66.

15. Krassioukov A, Warburton DE, Teasell R, et al. A systematic review of the management of autonomic dysreflexia after spinal cord injury. Arch Phys Med Rehabil 2009;90(4):682–95.

16. Bristow S, Dalal K, Santos JO, et al. Prevalence of hypertension, dyslipidemia, and diabetes mellitus after spinal cord injury. Fed Pract 2013;15–8.

17. Ravensbergen HR, Lear SA, Claydon VE. Waist circumference is the best index for obesity-related cardiovascular disease risk in individuals with spinal cord injury. J Neurotrauma 2013;31:292–300.

18. Laughton G, Buchholz A, Ginis KM, et al. Lowering body mass index cutoffs better identifies obese persons with spinal cord injury. Spinal Cord 2009;47(10): 757–62.

19. U.S. Department of Agriculture, U.S. Department of Health and Human Services. Dietary guidelines for Americans, 2010. Washington, DC: Government Printing Office; 2010.

20. Goldstein DJ. Beneficial health effects of modest weight loss. Int J Obes Relat Metab Disord 1992;16(6):397–415.

21. Mertens IL, Van Gaal LF. Overweight, obesity, and blood pressure: the effects of modest weight reduction. Obes Res 2000;8(3):270–8.

22. Pentland WE, Twomey LT. Upper limb function in persons with long term paraplegia and implications for independence: Part II. Paraplegia 1994;32(4): 219–24.

23. Van Drongelen S, Van der Woude LH, Janssen TW, et al. Mechanical load on the upper extremity during wheelchair activities. Arch Phys Med Rehabil 2005; 86(6):1214–20.

24. Nash MS, van de Ven I, van Elk N, et al. Effects of circuit resistance training on fitness attributes and upper-extremity pain in middle-aged men with paraplegia. Arch Phys Med Rehabil 2007;88(1):70–5.

25. Beavers KM, Lyles MF, Davis CC, et al. Is lost lean mass from intentional weight loss recovered during weight regain in postmenopausal women? Am J Clin Nutr 2011;94(3):767–74.

26. Chaston TB, Dixon JB, O'Brien PE. Changes in fat-free mass during significant weight loss: a systematic review. Int J Obes (Lond) 2007;31(5):743–50.

27. Villareal DT, Chode S, Parimi N, et al. Weight loss, exercise, or both and physical function in obese older adults. N Engl J Med 2011;364(13):1218–29.

28. Nash MS, Cowan RE, Kressler J. Evidence-based and heuristic approaches for customization of care in cardiometabolic syndrome after spinal cord injury. J Spinal Cord Med 2012;35(5):278–92.

29. Feasel S, Suzanne LG. The impact of diet on cardiovascular disease risk in individuals with spinal cord injury. Top Spinal Cord Inj Rehabil 2009;14(3):56–68.

30. Levine AM, Nash MS, Green BA, et al. An examination of dietary intakes and nutritional status of chronic healthy spinal cord injured individuals. Paraplegia 1992;30(12):880–9.

31. United States Department of Agriculture. SuperTracker. 2013:1. Available at: https://www.supertracker.usda.gov/default.aspx.

32. Buchholz AC, McGillivray CF, Pencharz PB. Differences in resting metabolic rate between paraplegic and able-bodied subjects are explained by differences in body composition. Am J Clin Nutr 2003;77(2):371–8.

33. Monroe MB, Tataranni PA, Pratley R, et al. Lower daily energy expenditure as measured by a respiratory chamber in subjects with spinal cord injury compared with control subjects. Am J Clin Nutr 1998;68(6):1223–7.

34. Tanhoffer RA, Tanhoffer AI, Raymond J, et al. Comparison of methods to assess energy expenditure and physical activity in people with spinal cord injury. J Spinal Cord Med 2012;35(1):35–45.

35. Washburn RA, Zhu W, McAuley E, et al. The physical activity scale for individuals with physical disabilities: development and evaluation. Arch Phys Med Rehabil 2002;83(2):193–200.

36. Ginis KA, Latimer AE, Hicks AL, et al. Development and evaluation of an activity measure for people with spinal cord injury. Med Sci Sports Exerc 2005;37(7):1099–111.

37. Crovetti R, Porrini M, Santangelo A, et al. The influence of thermic effect of food on satiety. Eur J Clin Nutr 1998;52(7):482–8.

38. Raben A, Agerholm-Larsen L, Flint A, et al. Meals with similar energy densities but rich in protein, fat, carbohydrate, or alcohol have different effects on energy expenditure and substrate metabolism but not on appetite and energy intake. Am J Clin Nutr 2003;77(1):91–100.

39. Dulloo AG. The search for compounds that stimulate thermogenesis in obesity management: from pharmaceuticals to functional food ingredients. Obes Rev 2011;12(10):866–83.

40. Keogh JB, Lau CW, Noakes M, et al. Effects of meals with high soluble fibre, high amylose barley variant on glucose, insulin, satiety and thermic effect of food in healthy lean women. Eur J Clin Nutr 2007;61(5):597–604.

41. Konings E, Schoffelen PF, Stegen J, et al. Effect of polydextrose and soluble maize fibre on energy metabolism, metabolic profile and appetite control in overweight men and women. Br J Nutr 2014;111:111–21.

42. Poppitt SD, Livesey G, Elia M. Energy expenditure and net substrate utilization in men ingesting usual and high amounts of nonstarch polysaccharide. Am J Clin Nutr 1998;68(4):820–6.

43. Raben A, Christensen NJ, Madsen J, et al. Decreased postprandial thermogenesis and fat oxidation but increased fullness after a high-fiber meal compared with a low-fiber meal. Am J Clin Nutr 1994;59(6):1386–94.

44. Gruendel S, Garcia AL, Otto B, et al. Carob pulp preparation rich in insoluble dietary fiber and polyphenols enhances lipid oxidation and lowers postprandial acylated ghrelin in humans. J Nutr 2006;136(6):1533–8.

45. Howarth NC, Saltzman E, Roberts SB. Dietary fiber and weight regulation. Nutr Rev 2001;59(5):129–39.

46. Wisker E, Maltz A, Feldheim W. Metabolizable energy of diets low or high in dietary fiber from cereals when eaten by humans. J Nutr 1988;118(8):945–52.

47. Alexander LR, Spungen AM, Liu MH, et al. Resting metabolic rate in subjects with paraplegia: the effect of pressure sores. Arch Phys Med Rehabil 1995;76(9):819–22.

48. Cox SA, Weiss SM, Posuniak EA, et al. Energy expenditure after spinal cord injury: an evaluation of stable rehabilitating patients. J Trauma 1985;25(5):419–23.

49. Gorgey AS, Chiodo AE, Zemper ED, et al. Relationship of spasticity to soft tissue body composition and the metabolic profile in persons with chronic motor complete spinal cord injury. J Spinal Cord Med 2010;33(1):6–15.

50. Liusuwan A, Widman L, Abresch RT, et al. Altered body composition affects resting energy expenditure and interpretation of body mass index in children with spinal cord injury. J Spinal Cord Med 2004;27(Suppl 1):S24–8.

51. Yamasaki M, Irizawa M, Komura T, et al. Daily energy expenditure in active and inactive persons with spinal cord injury. J Hum Ergol (Tokyo) 1992;21(2):125–33.

52. Bauman WA, Spungen AM, Wang J, et al. The relationship between energy expenditure and lean tissue in monozygotic twins discordant for spinal cord injury. J Rehabil Res Dev 2004;41(1):1–8.

53. Lee M, Zhu W, Hedrick B, et al. Determining metabolic equivalent values of physical activities for persons with paraplegia. Disabil Rehabil 2010;32(4): 336–43.

54. Sedlock DA, Laventure SJ. Body composition and resting energy expenditure in long term spinal cord injury. Paraplegia 1990;28(7):448–54.

55. Yilmaz B, Yasar E, Goktepe S, et al. Basal metabolic rate and autonomic nervous system dysfunction in men with spinal cord injury. Obesity (Silver Spring) 2007;15(11):2683–7.

56. Spungen AM, Bauman WA, Wang J, et al. The relationship between total body potassium and resting energy expenditure in individuals with paraplegia. Arch Phys Med Rehabil 1993;74(9):965–8.

57. Mollinger LA, Spurr GB, el Ghatit AZ, et al. Daily energy expenditure and basal metabolic rates of patients with spinal cord injury. Arch Phys Med Rehabil 1985; 66(7):420–6.

58. Dionyssiotis Y. Malnutrition in spinal cord injury: more than nutritional deficiency. J Clin Med Res 2012;4(4):227.

59. Groah SL, Nash MS, Ljungberg IH, et al. Nutrient intake and body habitus after spinal cord injury: an analysis by sex and level of injury. J Spinal Cord Med 2009;32(1):25–33.

60. Perret C, Stoffel-Kurt N. Comparison of nutritional intake between individuals with acute and chronic spinal cord injury. J Spinal Cord Med 2011;34(6):569–75.

61. Tomey KM, Chen DM, Wang X, et al. Dietary intake and nutritional status of urban community-dwelling men with paraplegia. Arch Phys Med Rehabil 2005; 86(4):664–71.

62. Aquilani R, Boschi F, Contardi A, et al. Energy expenditure and nutritional adequacy of rehabilitation paraplegics with asymptomatic bacteriuria and pressure sores. Spinal Cord 2001;39(8):437–41.

63. Sabour H, Javidan AN, Vafa MR, et al. Calorie and macronutrients intake in people with spinal cord injuries: an analysis by sex and injury-related variables. Nutrition 2012;28(2):143–7.

64. Moussavi RM, Ribas-Cardus F, Rintala DH, et al. Dietary and serum lipids in individuals with spinal cord injury living in the community. J Rehabil Res Dev 2001; 38(2):225–33.

65. Battista P, Di Primio R, Di Luzio A, et al. Correlations between dietetic fiber and serum levels of total cholesterol and HDL-cholesterol. Boll Soc Ital Biol Sper 1983;59(1):83–6.

66. Brown L, Rosner B, Willett WW, et al. Cholesterol-lowering effects of dietary fiber: a meta-analysis. Am J Clin Nutr 1999;69(1):30–42.

67. Mietus-Snyder ML, Shigenaga MK, Suh JH, et al. A nutrient-dense, high-fiber, fruit-based supplement bar increases HDL cholesterol, particularly large HDL, lowers homocysteine, and raises glutathione in a 2-wk trial. FASEB J 2012;26:3515–27.

68. Reyna-Villasmil N, Bermudez-Pirela V, Mengual-Moreno E, et al. Oat-derived beta-glucan significantly improves HDLC and diminishes LDLC and non-HDL cholesterol in overweight individuals with mild hypercholesterolemia. Am J Ther 2007;14(2):203–12.

69. Walters JL, Buchholz AC, Martin Ginis KA, et al. Evidence of dietary inadequacy in adults with chronic spinal cord injury. Spinal Cord 2009;47(4):318–22.

70. Cameron KJ, Nyulasi IB, Collier GR, et al. Assessment of the effect of increased dietary fibre intake on bowel function in patients with spinal cord injury. Spinal Cord 1996;34(5):277–83.

71. Krassioukov A, Eng JJ, Claxton G, et al. Neurogenic bowel management after spinal cord injury: a systematic review of the evidence. Spinal Cord 2010; 48(10):718–33.

72. Lam T, Chen Z, Sayed-Ahmed M, et al. Potential role of oxidative stress on the prescription of rehabilitation interventions in spinal cord injury. Spinal Cord 2013; 51:656–62.

73. Gerrior S, Bente L. Nutrient content of the US food supply, 1909–1999. Center for Nutrition Policy and Promotion, U.S. Department of Agriculture; 2002.

74. Tomita LY, Roteli-Martins CM, Villa LL, et al. Associations of dietary dark-green and deep-yellow vegetables and fruits with cervical intraepithelial neoplasia: modification by smoking. Br J Nutr 2011;105(6):928.

75. Office of Dietary Supplements, National Institutes of Health. Dietary Supplement Fact Sheet: Vitamin A. 2011;2013(12/09):1.

76. Office of Dietary Supplements, National Institutes of Health. Dietary Supplement Fact Sheet: Vitamin D. 2011;2013(12/09):1. Available at: http://ods.od.nih.gov/factsheets/VitaminD-HealthProfessional/.

77. Office of Dietary Supplements, National Institutes of Health. Dietary Supplement Fact Sheet: Vitamin E. 2013;2013(12/09):1. Available at: http://ods.od.nih.gov/factsheets/VitaminE-HealthProfessional/.

78. Office of Dietary Supplements, National Institutes of Health. Dietary Supplement Fact Sheet: Vitamin C. 2013;2013(12/09). Available at: http://ods.od.nih.gov/factsheets/VitaminC-HealthProfessional/.

79. University of Maryland Medical Center. Viamin H (biotin). 2013;2013(12/09):1. Available at: http://umm.edu/health/medical/altmed/supplement/vitamin-h-biotin.

80. MedlinePlus. Pantothenic acid (Vitamin B5). 2012;2013(12/09):1. Available at: http://www.nlm.nih.gov/medlineplus/druginfo/natural/853.htm.

81. Oldenburg O, Kribben A, Baumgart D, et al. Treatment of orthostatic hypotension. Curr Opin Pharmacol 2002;2(6):740–7.

82. Krassioukov A, Claydon VE. The clinical problems in cardiovascular control following spinal cord injury: an overview. Prog Brain Res 2006;152:223–9.

83. Sacks FM, Svetkey LP, Vollmer WM, et al. Effects on blood pressure of reduced dietary sodium and the dietary approaches to stop hypertension (DASH) diet. N Engl J Med 2001;344(1):3–10.

84. Kastorini C, Milionis HJ, Esposito K, et al. The effect of Mediterranean diet on metabolic syndrome and its components: a meta-analysis of 50 studies and 534,906 individuals. J Am Coll Cardiol 2011;57(11):1299–313.

85. World Health Organization. Global strategy on diet, physical activity and health. WHO Prevention of Noncommunicable Diseases (PND) Noncommunicable Diseases and Mental Health: Geneva, Switzerland; 2013.

86. U.S. Department of Health and Human Services, Center for Disease Control and Prevention. Physical Activity Guidelines for Americans. 2011. Available at: http://www.cdc.gov/physicalactivity/everyone/guidelines/adults.html.

87. American College of Sports Medicine (ACSM) and the American Medical Association (AMA). Exercise is Medicine Health Care Providers' Action Guide. 2008;2013. Available at: http://exerciseismedicine.org/documents/HCPAction Guide.pdf.

88. SCIAction Canada. Physical activity guidelines for adults with spinal cord injury. Hamilton, Ontario: McMaster University; 2011.

89. Kressler J, Burns P, Betancourt L, et al. Circuit training and protein supplementation in persons with chronic tetraplegia. Med Sci Sports Exerc 2014. [Epub ahead of print].

90. Hicks AL, Martin KA, Ditor DS, et al. Long-term exercise training in persons with spinal cord injury: effects on strength, arm ergometry performance and psychological well-being. Spinal Cord 2003;41(1):34–43.

91. Haisma J, Van der Woude L, Stam H, et al. Physical capacity in wheelchair-dependent persons with a spinal cord injury: a critical review of the literature. Spinal Cord 2006;44(11):642–52.

92. Spungen AM, Wang J, Pierson RN Jr, et al. Soft tissue body composition differences in monozygotic twins discordant for spinal cord injury. J Appl Physiol (1985) 2000;88(4):1310–5.

93. West CR, Wong SC, Krassioukov AV. Autonomic cardiovascular control in Paralympic athletes with spinal cord injury. Med Sci Sports Exerc 2013;46:60–8.

94. Price M. Energy expenditure and metabolism during exercise in persons with a spinal cord injury. Sports Med 2010;40(8):681–96.

95. Donnelly J, Blair S, Jakicic J, et al. American College of Sports Medicine Position Stand. Appropriate physical activity intervention strategies for weight loss and prevention of weight regain for adults. Med Sci Sports Exerc 2009;41(2):459–71.

96. Weidinger KA, Lovegreen SL, Elliott MB, et al. How to make exercise counseling more effective: lessons from rural America. J Fam Pract 2008;57:394–402.

97. Letts L, Ginis KA, Faulkner G, et al. Preferred methods and messengers for delivering physical activity information to people with spinal cord injury: a focus group study. Rehabil Psychol 2011;56(2):128.

98. Bonninger M, Waters R, Chase T, et al. Preservation of upper limb function following spinal cord injury: a clinical practice guideline for health-care professionals. J Spinal Cord Med 2005;28:434–70.

99. American College of Sports Medicine. ACSM ProFinder. 2013. Available at: http://certification.acsm.org/pro-finder.

100. Ballinger DA, Rintala DH, Hart KA. The relation of shoulder pain and range-of-motion problems to functional limitations, disability, and perceived health of men with spinal cord injury: a multifaceted longitudinal study. Arch Phys Med Rehabil 2000;81(12):1575–81.

101. Subbarao JV, Klopfstein J, Turpin R. Prevalence and impact of wrist and shoulder pain in patients with spinal cord injury. J Spinal Cord Med 1995;18(1):9–13.

102. Curtis K, Tyner T, Zachary L, et al. Effect of a standard exercise protocol on shoulder pain in long-term wheelchair users. Spinal Cord 1999;37(6):421–9.

103. Nawoczenski DA, Ritter-Soronen JM, Wilson CM, et al. Clinical trial of exercise for shoulder pain in chronic spinal injury. Phys Ther 2006;86(12):1604–18.

104. American College of Cardiology (ACC)/American Heart Association (AHA) Task Force. ACC/AHA Joint Guidelines. 2013. Available at: http://my.americanheart. org/professional/StatementsGuidelines/ByTopic/TopicsA-C/ACCAHA-Joint-Guidelines_UCM_321694_Article.jsp.

105. National Institute of Diabetes and Digestive and Kidney Diseases (NIDDK). Diabetes Prevention Program (DPP). 2013. Available at: http://diabetes.niddk.nih. gov/dm/pubs/preventionprogram/.

106. Orchard M, Fowler S, Temprosa M. Impact of intensive lifestyle and metformin therapy on cardiovascular disease risk factors in the diabetes prevention program. Diabetes Care 2005;28(4):888–94.

107. Knowler WC, Fowler SE, Hamman RF, et al. 10-year follow-up of diabetes incidence and weight loss in the Diabetes Prevention Program Outcomes Study. Lancet 2009;374(9702):1677–86.

108. Brenes G, Dearwater S, Shapera R, et al. High density lipoprotein cholesterol concentrations in physically active and sedentary spinal cord injured patients. Arch Phys Med Rehabil 1986;67(7):445–50.

109. Zlotolow SP, Levy E, Bauman WA. The serum lipoprotein profile in veterans with paraplegia: the relationship to nutritional factors and body mass index. J Am Paraplegia Soc 1992;15(3):158–62.

110. Karlsson A, Attvall S, Jansson P, et al. Influence of the sympathetic nervous system on insulin sensitivity and adipose tissue metabolism: a study in spinal cord—injured subjects. Metabolism 1995;44(1):52–8.

111. Maki KC, Briones ER, Langbein WE, et al. Associations between serum lipids and indicators of adiposity in men with spinal cord injury. Paraplegia 1995; 33(2):102–9.

112. McGlinchey-Berroth R, Morrow L, Ahlquist M, et al. Late-life spinal cord injury and aging with a long term injury: characteristics of two emerging populations. J Spinal Cord Med 1995;18(3):183–93.

113. Bauman WA, Kahn NN, Grimm DR, et al. Risk factors for atherogenesis and cardiovascular autonomic function in persons with spinal cord injury. Spinal Cord 1999;37(9):601–16.

114. Washburn RA, Figoni SF. High density lipoprotein cholesterol in individuals with spinal cord injury: the potential role of physical activity. Spinal Cord 1999;37(10): 685–95.

115. Bauman WA, Spungen AM. Carbohydrate and lipid metabolism in chronic spinal cord injury. J Spinal Cord Med 2001;24(4):266–77.

116. Wahman K, Nash MS, Lewis JE, et al. Cardiovascular disease risk and the need for prevention after paraplegia determined by conventional multifactorial risk models: the Stockholm spinal cord injury study. J Rehabil Med 2011; 43(3):237–42.

117. Spungen AM, Adkins RH, Stewart CA, et al. Factors influencing body composition in persons with spinal cord injury: a cross-sectional study. J Appl Physiol (1985) 2003;95(6):2398–407.

118. Gorgey AS, Gater DR. A preliminary report on the effects of the level of spinal cord injury on the association between central adiposity and metabolic profile. PM R 2011;3(5):440–6.

119. Liang H, Chen D, Wang Y, et al. Different risk factor patterns for metabolic syndrome in men with spinal cord injury compared with able-bodied men despite similar prevalence rates. Arch Phys Med Rehabil 2007;88(9):1198–204.

120. Post M, Van Leeuwen C. Psychosocial issues in spinal cord injury: a review. Spinal Cord 2012;50(5):382–9.

121. Mehta S, Orenczuk S, Hansen KT, et al. An evidence-based review of the effectiveness of cognitive behavioral therapy for psychosocial issues post-spinal cord injury. Rehabil Psychol 2011;56(1):15.

122. Cowan R, Nash M, Anderson K. Exercise participation barrier prevalence and association with exercise participation status in individuals with spinal cord injury. Spinal Cord 2012;51(1):27–32.

123. Cowan RE, Nash MS, Anderson-Erisman K. Perceived exercise barriers and odds of exercise participation among persons with SCI living in high-income households. Top Spinal Cord Inj Rehabil 2012;18(2):126–7.

124. Wong S, Graham A, Grimble G, et al. Spinal clinic for obese out-patient project (SCOOP)—a 1 year report. Food Nutr 2011;2:901–7.

125. Jacobs KA, Burns P, Kressler J, et al. Heavy reliance on carbohydrate across a wide range of exercise intensities during voluntary arm ergometry in persons with paraplegia. J Spinal Cord Med 2013;36:427–35.

126. Kressler J, Nash MS, Burns PA, et al. Metabolic responses to four different body weight supported locomotor training approaches in persons with incomplete spinal cord injury. Arch Phys Med Rehabil 2013;94:1436–42.

127. Burns P, Kressler J, Nash MS. Physiological responses to exergaming after spinal cord injury. Top Spinal Cord Inj Rehabil 2012;18(4):331–9.

128. Kressler J, Cowan RE, Ginnity K, et al. Subjective measures of exercise intensity to gauge substrate partitioning in persons with paraplegia. Top Spinal Cord Inj Rehabil 2012;18(3):205–11.

129. American Diabetes Association. Diagnosis and classification of diabetes mellitus. Diabetes Care 2010;33(Suppl 1):S62–9.

130. American Diabetes Association. Diagnosis and classification of diabetes mellitus. Diabetes Care 2013;36(Suppl 1):S67–74.

131. Goldberg RB. Guideline-driven intervention on sci-associated dyslipidemia, metabolic syndrome, and glucose intolerance using pharmacological agents. Top Spinal Cord Inj Rehabil 2009;14(3):46–57.

132. Bennett WL, Odelola OA, Wilson LM, et al. Evaluation of guideline recommendations on oral medications for type 2 diabetes mellitus a systematic review. Ann Intern Med 2012;156(1 Pt 1):27–36.

133. Nash MS, Kressler J, Betancourt L, et al. Salsalate improves fasting and postprandial glycemic and lipid levels in persons with chronic tetraplegia. Top Spinal Cord Inj Rehabil 2013;19:2.

134. National Cholesterol Education Program (NCEP) Expert Panel on Detection, Evaluation, and Treatment of High Blood Cholesterol in Adults (Adult Treatment Panel III). Third report of the National Cholesterol Education Program (NCEP) expert panel on detection, evaluation, and treatment of high blood cholesterol in adults (Adult Treatment Panel III) final report. Circulation 2002;106(25): 3143–421.

135. Dyson-Hudson TA, Nash MS. Guideline-driven assessment of cardiovascular disease and related risks after spinal cord injury. Top Spinal Cord Inj Rehabil 2009;14(3):32–45.

136. Stone NJ, Robinson J, Lichtenstein AH, et al. 2013 ACC/AHA guideline on the treatment of blood cholesterol to reduce atherosclerotic cardiovascular risk in adults a report of the American College of Cardiology/American Heart Association task force on practice guidelines. J Am Coll Cardiol 2013. [Epub ahead of print].

137. Nash MS, Johnson BM, Jacobs PL. Combined hyperlipidemia in a single subject with tetraplegia: ineffective risk reduction after atorvastatin monotherapy. J Spinal Cord Med 2004;27(5):484–7.

138. Thompson PD, Clarkson P, Karas RH. Statin-associated myopathy. JAMA 2003; 289(13):1681–90.
139. Goldberg AC. Clinical trial experience with extended-release niacin (Niaspan): dose-escalation study. Am J Cardiol 1998;82(12):35U–8U.
140. Morgan JM, Capuzzi DM, Guyton JR. A new extended-release niacin (Niaspan): efficacy, tolerability, and safety in hypercholesterolemic patients. Am J Cardiol 1998;82(12):29U–34U.
141. Guyton JR, Goldberg AC, Kreisberg RA, et al. Effectiveness of once-nightly dosing of extended-release niacin alone and in combination for hypercholesterolemia. Am J Cardiol 1998;82(6):737–43.
142. Nash MS, Lewis JE, Dyson-Hudson TA, et al. Safety, tolerance, and efficacy of extended-release niacin monotherapy for treating dyslipidemia risks in persons with chronic tetraplegia: a randomized multicenter controlled trial. Arch Phys Med Rehabil 2011;92(3):399–410.
143. Chobanian AV, Bakris GL, Black HR, et al. Seventh report of the Joint National Committee on Prevention, Detection, Evaluation, and Treatment of High Blood Pressure. Hypertension 2003;42(6):1206–52.
144. Jennings HR, Cook TS. Hypertension: clinical practice updates. Lenexa, KS: American College of Clinical Pharmacy (ACCP); 2010. p. 7–20.
145. Yates AA, Schlicker SA, Suitor CW. Dietary reference intakes: the new basis for recommendations for calcium and related nutrients, B vitamins, and choline. J Am Diet Assoc 1998;98(6):699–706.
146. Ross AC, Taylor CL, Yaktine AL, et al. Dietary reference intakes for calcium and vitamin D. Washington, DC: National Academies Press; 2010.
147. Cranney A, Horsley T, O'Donnell S, et al. Effectiveness and safety of vitamin D in relation to bone health. Rockville, MD: US Department of Health and Human Services, Public Health Service, Agency for Healthcare Research and Quality; 2007.
148. Bassett-Gunter RL, Martin Ginis KA, Latimer-Cheung AE. Do you want the good news or the bad news? Gain-versus loss-framed messages following health risk information: the effects on leisure time physical activity beliefs and cognitions. Health Psychol 2013;32:1188–98.

Strategies for Prevention of Urinary Tract Infections in Neurogenic Bladder Dysfunction

Lance L. Goetz, MD*, Adam P. Klausner, MD

KEYWORDS

- Spinal cord injuries • Neurogenic bladder • Urinary tract infection
- Catheter-associated urinary tract infection (CAUTI)

KEY POINTS

- Urinary tract infection (UTI) is a clinical diagnosis, and treatment depends on the presence and severity of symptoms.
- Providers should not treat asymptomatic bacteriuria, and pyuria alone may not be an indication for treatment.
- Because of an increased incidence of resistant bacterial species in persons with spinal cord injury and disorders (SCI & D), urine culture should be obtained before the initiation of antibiotic therapy.
- Urodynamic evaluation is the standard of care to ensure safe bladder function, and intermittent catheterization is the preferred bladder management.
- Mechanical strategies for the prevention of UTIs in persons with SCI & D include use of hydrophilic, closed-system, and antibiotic-coated catheters as well as bladder irrigation and fluid restriction.
- Medical strategies for the prevention of UTIs in persons with SCI & D include antibiotic prophylaxis, cranberry compounds, D-mannose, methenamine, urinary acidifiers, and bacterial interference.

INTRODUCTION

Neurogenic bladder is a common and distressing complication of spinal cord injury and disorders (SCI & D). Individuals with neurogenic bladder dysfunction are often unable to completely empty their urinary bladders. As a result, many of these individuals must perform clean intermittent catheterization (CIC) or use indwelling urinary catheters. Use of urinary catheters is associated with high rates of urinary tract infections

Department of Veterans Affairs, Hunter Holmes McGuire VA Medical Center, 1201 Broad Rock Boulevard, Richmond, VA 23249, USA
* Corresponding author.
E-mail address: lance.goetz@va.gov

Phys Med Rehabil Clin N Am 25 (2014) 605–618
http://dx.doi.org/10.1016/j.pmr.2014.04.002
1047-9651/14/$ – see front matter Published by Elsevier Inc.

pmr.theclinics.com

(UTIs), termed catheter-associated UTIs (CAUTI). UTIs remain the most frequent type of infection in persons with SCI & D, with an average of 2.5 episodes per year.[1,2]

Before World War II, urinary tract complications were considered to be the number 1 cause of death in the acute period after SCI. However, advances in urologic diagnosis and management through the use of urodynamic assessments and CIC have reduced acute deaths and complications, improving the urinary tract–related quality of life for persons with SCI & D. Despite these advances, morbidity from UTIs remains common. In this regard, optimal urinary tract management is critical not only for the prevention of complications and illnesses but for the optimal social integration of the person with SCI & D.

This article is not intended to provide an exhaustive review of neurogenic bladder dysfunction after SCI & D, because detailed reviews of neurogenic bladder dysfunction have previously been published[3,4] Rather, the objectives of the article are to: (1) define the problem of UTIs after SCI & D, (2) discuss the relationship of bladder management to UTIs, (3) describe mechanical strategies for UTI prevention in SCI & D, and (4) describe medical strategies for UTI prevention in SCI & D. The reader is also referred to the detailed guideline by Hooton and colleagues,[5] which details evidence and recommendations regarding practices for prevention of CAUTI.

THE PROBLEM OF UTIS AFTER SCI & D
Bacteriuria

The definitions of what represents significant bacteriuria vary. Investigators and clinicians frequently define infection based on bacteriuria levels ranging from 10^3 to 10^5 colony-forming units (CFU) per milliliter of urine. However, insufficient data exist to recommend a standardized level for the diagnosis of CAUTI.[5] Historically, the medical literature pertaining to urinary catheters has not made clear distinctions between asymptomatic bacteriuria and UTI. Often the term UTI has been used when bacteriuria (with or without symptoms) is present.[5] The key problem, then, is that persons with SCI & D who use urinary catheters commonly have bacteriuria. The standard of care among SCI & D providers is not to treat asymptomatic bacteriuria, which has been defined as 10^5 CFU of 1 or more organisms in an appropriately collected specimen in an asymptomatic person,[5] with antibiotics.

Pyuria

Pyuria, defined as white blood cells (WBC) in the urine, is also commonly seen in individuals with neurogenic bladder dysfunction and especially in catheterized patients. However, in the catheterized patient, pyuria alone is not diagnostic of either asymptomatic bacteriuria or CAUTI.[1,5] Different researchers have defined significant pyuria variably, with levels as low as 5 WBC per high-powered field being considered clinically significant. However, there is disagreement regarding a threshold for significant pyuria, because many persons with SCI & D have chronic pyuria but no overt signs of illness (eg, fevers, chills, nausea, vomiting).

Bacterial Colonization

Colonization of the bladder with bacteriuria is the norm in persons with SCI & D who use urinary catheters, either indwelling or intermittent.[1,6] As noted earlier, treatment with antibiotics is not justified based on the presence of bacteriuria alone. Because of the risk of recurrent infections and development of resistant organisms in individuals with SCI & D, urine cultures should be obtained before initiation of antibiotic therapy in symptomatic persons. Empirical therapy may then be initiated with the opportunity of adjusting antimicrobial therapy based on culture results.

UTI Symptoms

The differentiation between asymptomatic bacterial colonization and clinical UTI can be difficult and is compounded by a lack of consensus regarding what constitutes UTI symptoms, the combination of symptoms and laboratory findings necessary for the diagnosis, and the symptoms that require antibiotic treatment (vs being managed with conservative measures, such as increasing fluid intake or catheterizations). UTI symptoms in individuals with SCI & D are diverse in both type and severity. These symptoms may include fever, rigors, chills, nausea and vomiting, abdominal discomfort, sweating, muscular spasms, fatigue, and autonomic dysreflexia (AD). Individuals may also present with cloudy or malodorous urine, increased urinary sediment, and catheter blockage. However, typical presenting symptoms experienced by individuals without SCI & D, such as dysuria, urinary frequency, and urinary urgency, may be absent.

As discussed further later, there is a need for consistency of reporting of various signs and symptoms of UTI. This factor has led to the development of clinical data sets to facilitate this process.[7] Signs and symptoms vary in their usefulness for UTI diagnosis. Massa and colleagues[8] reported that cloudy urine had the highest accuracy (83.1%) and leukocytes in the urine had the highest sensitivity (82.8%) for the presence of UTI. Fever had very high specificity (99%) but very low sensitivity (6.9%). In addition, AD was found to be both insensitive and nonspecific, because AD may be triggered by multiple causes. Other symptoms, including kidney/bladder discomfort, increased spasticity, feeling sick, sense of unease, increased need to perform catheterization, feeling tired, incontinence, and foul-smelling urine, all had high sensitivity (77%–95%) but very low specificity (<50%). Persons with SCI & D are not always able to accurately predict the presence of a UTI based on their symptoms.[9]

UTI Diagnosis

A UTI is characterized by the new onset of symptoms and not merely the presence of bacteria or WBC in the urine. To make the diagnosis, relevant laboratory findings, including bacteriuria (seen on urinalysis, dipstick, or culture), pyuria (leukocyturia), or a positive urine culture, must be accompanied by symptoms (see earlier section).[10] In individuals with neurogenic bladder dysfunction, asymptomatic bacteriuria of varying degrees is the norm.[1] Persons with SCI & D often do not present with similar symptoms to those in the general population, because of impaired or absent pain sensation.

Data Sets and Consensus Statements

Interpretation of UTI signs and symptoms is not standardized across systems of care or in different regions of the world. Led by Biering-Sorenson and colleagues,[11] international data sets for SCI & D have been developed. Recently, a basic data set for UTI was developed to standardize collection and reporting of the minimal amount of information required to define a possible UTI in daily practice.[7] This data set also makes it possible to evaluate and compare the results from various published studies. The importance of the urinary tract in SCI & D is evident in that data sets have been developed not only for UTI but also lower urinary tract function, imaging, and urodynamics.[12–14] Data sets are incorporated into the National Institute of Neurological Disorders and Stroke common data elements to facilitate sharing of data from different studies.[15]

THE RELATIONSHIP OF BLADDER MANAGEMENT TO UTIS
Neurourology

There is tremendous complexity in the functioning of both the bladder and external urethral sphincter as distinct anatomic and functional units. However, the key to their proper functioning is the process through which these organs work together in a tightly orchestrated and reciprocal fashion. Thus, for effective urine storage to occur, the bladder must be in a state of relaxation while the external urethral sphincter is simultaneously in a state of tight contraction. Alternatively, when the voiding phase is initiated, a specific sequence of events needs to occur: first, the urethral sphincter relaxes, and then, the bladder contracts. This coordinated reciprocal control of the bladder and the external urethral sphincter is mediated by a control center in the brainstem called the pontine micturition center (PMC).[16]

Accordingly, any neurologic injury above the PMC leads to suppression of inhibitory inputs from higher cortical centers and results in neurogenic detrusor overactivity with intact coordination of the external urethral sphincter and bladder. Injuries to the spinal cord below the PMC but above the sacral motor outflow result in neurogenic detrusor overactivity with a lack of external urethral sphincter and bladder coordination, a condition known as detrusor sphincter dyssynergia. This is the situation seen in most individuals who have complete (American Spinal Injury Association Impairment Scale A) suprasacral spinal cord injury. The problem in this situation is that the lack of coordination can lead to sustained high pressures in the bladder, with corresponding increases in complications, including UTIs, vesicoureteral reflux, calculi, hydronephrosis, and kidney damage.[16] Thus, knowing some basic neurourology and the main location of a neurologic injury, the likely form of neurogenic bladder dysfunction can be predicted. Forms of neurogenic bladder dysfunction and descriptions based on location of neurologic injury are presented in **Table 1** according to the functional model of voiding dysfunction originally described by Wein.[17,18]

Bladder Management in Neurogenic Bladder Dysfunction

As described earlier, an understanding of the lower urinary tract pathophysiology in an individual with neurogenic bladder dysfunction is key to developing an optimized plan for long-term bladder management. The goal is to ensure complete bladder emptying before the occurrence of high-pressure, uncoordinated involuntary detrusor contractions. Thus, when patients or clinicians ask about the correct time

Table 1
A simple classification of neurogenic bladder dysfunction[a]

	Condition
Sphincter function	
Too loose	Neurogenic incompetent urethral closure mechanism
Too tight	Detrusor sphincter dyssynergia
Bladder function	
Underactive	Neurogenic detrusor acontractility
Overactive	Neurogenic detrusor overactivity
Injury location	
Above the PMC	Neurogenic detrusor overactivity
Below the PMC and above SMO (S2–4)	Neurogenic detrusor overactivity with detrusor sphincter dyssynergia
At or below SMO (S2–4)	Detrusor acontractility with or without incompetent urethral closure mechanism

Abbreviations: PMC, pontine micturition center; SMO, sacral motor outflow.
[a] Based on the functional model of voiding dysfunction by Wein.[17,18]

interval for the performance of CIC, these individuals should be redirected to think about bladder management in terms of appropriate volume intervals. Volume intervals are best determined through the use of a well-performed urodynamics evaluation.

The urodynamic study should be performed in all individuals with neurogenic bladder dysfunction as soon as stable bladder functioning has been achieved, and again, when there is a change in clinical urologic status.[16] For example, an individual who has been performing CIC for 5 years without complications does not specifically need a new urodynamics test, because the risks of testing (stricture formation, infections) do not justify the small anticipated benefit. On the other hand, individuals with neurogenic bladder dysfunction who report increased rates of UTIs, difficulty catheterizing, leakage between catheterizations, development of new urinary calculi, hydronephrosis, or deterioration in renal function would clearly benefit from a repeat urodynamics test, because the cause of many of these conditions may be improper bladder management.

The urodynamics test involves placement of a urinary catheter and a rectal catheter to simultaneously measure bladder and intra-abdominal pressures.[16] The bladder is then infused with sterile saline at a defined rate to rapidly reproduce the filling-voiding cycle. During the filling phase, the compliance (elasticity) of the bladder can be calculated. Several studies have shown that poor compliance (equivalent to high stiffness) is associated with greater rates of upper tract deterioration and other urologic complications.[19,20] The presence, pressures, and volume at which any involuntary bladder contractions occur are recorded. The voiding phase is analyzed by simultaneously recording the urinary flow rate and the detrusor pressure. These data are then plotted on to various nomograms such as the International Continence Society nomogram. This strategy allows the urodynamicist to determine if the voiding cycle is obstructed (defined as high bladder pressures in the presence of a low urinary flow rate) or unobstructed. The patient's clinical history, pattern of pressure data, and the simultaneous collection of sphincter electromyographic activity and fluoroscopic images helps the urodynamicist determine the likely cause of neurogenic bladder dysfunction. For example, bladder outlet obstruction in a 25-year-old man with complete suprasacral spinal cord injury is likely caused by detrusor sphincter dyssynergia. Similar obstruction in an elderly man without known neurologic disease is most likely caused by benign prostatic hyperplasia.

Based on the results of the urodynamics test in conjunction with recommended annual studies, including upper tract imaging with a renal/bladder ultrasonography and laboratory tests to evaluate bladder function, a plan for bladder management is developed and implemented. Effective implementation of a bladder management plan likely includes a combination of behavioral modification (fluid restriction), pharmacotherapy, and CIC. Pharmacotherapy can be used to help suppress involuntary bladder contractions, increase bladder capacity, and lower bladder pressures. Second-line therapies, including injection of botulinum toxin, can be tried for refractory cases. Surgical diversions are available for the most severely affected individuals. Use of indwelling urinary catheters should be strongly discouraged because of high rates of infections and other severe complications. However, for some individuals, this option is the only available means to achieve bladder emptying.

Catheterization should be timed such that the bladder is emptied before the volume at which high-pressure involuntary contractions develop. A team approach is required, with necessary involvement from nurse educators, clinicians, occupational therapists, social workers, and family members/caregivers.[16] The bladder management plan is continually adjusted based on evolving patient needs and circumstances.

Recurrent UTIs in Individuals with Neurogenic Bladder Dysfunction

We would like to emphasize that many conditions such as recurrent UTIs are best controlled through the implementation of a well-designed bladder management plan. Therefore, patients with neurogenic bladder dysfunction who present with recurrent UTIs should first be treated by attempting to optimize their bladder management. In addition, a search for treatable sources of infection with imaging studies and cystourethroscopy should be implemented to identify treatable causes, including infected calculi, diverticuli, and strictures. However, after all available attempts have been exhausted, patients can be directed to use various preventive strategies, which is comprehensively reviewed in the following sections.

MECHANICAL STRATEGIES FOR UTI PREVENTION AFTER SCI & D

Several mechanical strategies have been developed to prevent UTIs in individuals who use urinary catheters. These strategies include use of sterile technique, closed-system kits, antibiotic-coated catheters, and changing of indwelling catheters on a more frequent basis. The following sections review the evidence for UTI prevention when using these strategies.

Intermittent Catheterization

Intermittent catheterization (IC), or intermittent self-catheterization, has become the standard of care for persons with SCI who have adequate hand function or caregiver support. IC may be performed using sterile technique, but clean technique, referred to as CIC, is more commonly used. IC should be performed every 4 to 6 hours. Persons with SCI & D using IC need to catheterize frequently enough to keep volumes lower than predetermined levels defined by urodynamic studies. Generally, the urodynamic goal is a storage pressure lower than 40 cm H_2O.[21] Future studies are needed to determine what factors influence the rate of UTIs in those who perform CIC.[22]

Catheter reuse
Reuse of catheters for IC is controversial and has never been approved by the US Food and Drug Administration for any catheter type. Many patients and providers argue that there is a theoretic increased infection risk. However, current evidence suggests that reuse after cleansing may be appropriate in certain circumstances.[23] In patients on IC, ascension of bacteria colonizing the urethra into the bladder is more likely to be the source of bacteriuria than introduction of new bacteria.[5] Rinsing with water, air-drying, microwaving, or soaking catheters in various agents are all effective in reducing bacteria on catheters. However, there are no published trials evaluating the effectiveness of any of these cleaning methods in preventing bacteriuria or CAUTI.[5]

Closed-system versus open-system catheters
There is no high-level evidence showing the superiority of sterile versus clean technique for reducing CAUTI. Likewise, evidence has not shown the superiority of closed or self-contained (also called no-touch) IC kits versus sterile technique. Use of the no-touch technique (in which the catheter and preattached collecting system are not touched by the patient) reduces microbial contamination of the catheter.[24] There is some evidence that use of sterile prepackaged catheter collection kits can reduce the frequency of UTIs in SCI.[23,25] However, these kits are expensive and must be justified to payers. They are generally tried only when an individual presents with recurrent UTIs. There is no catheterization technique that can be carried out without any risk of introducing organisms into the urinary tract.[1] It has been shown that most urethral

bacteria exist in the distal 15 mm of the urethra. This finding led to the development of intermittent catheter kits using an introducer tip to bypass the distal urethra, which was shown to decrease UTIs in hospitalized men with SCI & D.[26]

Hydrophilic catheters

Hydrophilic catheters have been developed with the goal of reducing friction and thereby reducing trauma during the catheterization process. De Ridder and colleagues,[27] in a randomized 1-year prospective trial in 2005, found a statistically significant reduction in UTIs with hydrophilic versus noncoated catheters. However, 64% of persons using hydrophilic catheters (vs 82% for noncoated catheters) still had 1 or more UTIs during the study period. Furthermore, there was no significant difference in bleeding, bacteriuria, or pyuria between the 2 groups. Stensballe and colleagues[28] found a reduction in hematuria and pain and higher patient preference for hydrophilic catheters. One study found no difference in the number of symptomatic UTIs versus noncoated catheters.[29] However, a more recent study by the same group[30] found that the use of a hydrophilic catheter reduced the risk of UTI in the acute period and significantly delayed the time to first UTI versus a plastic uncoated catheter. Hydrophilic catheters may also be useful for persons with urethral strictures or discomfort during catheterization.

External Catheters

Bladder management using an external catheter (also referred to as a condom or Texas catheter) is an option for some men with SCI & D. There is no effective equivalent option in common use for women. Some men with SCI & D use an external catheter to collect urine that leaks in between ICs; others use external catheters exclusively. Urodynamic evaluation is indicated to determine important variables such as the detrusor leak point pressure. Procedures to decrease bladder outlet resistance, including transurethral sphincterotomy and urethral stent placement, have been used in men with increased leak point pressures. Men with chronic suprasacral SCI & D using external catheters have more severe bladder trabeculation compared with other methods of bladder management.[31] In addition, it is important to recognize that penile retraction or abdominal obesity can make it difficult or impossible to maintain a proper fit with an external catheter. Furthermore, the use of external catheters does not prevent chronic bacterial colonization and pyuria. Residual urine with pyuria, worsening urinary retention, and hydronephrosis caused by increased pressure and poor emptying are all potential problems with external catheter usage.[32]

Indwelling Catheters

Persons with SCI & D who require indwelling catheters for long-term bladder management may nonetheless benefit from the addition of antimuscarinic medication. Use of the antimuscarinic oxybutynin in persons with SCI & D and chronic indwelling catheters has been associated with better bladder compliance and less hydronephrosis.[33] Suprapubic indwelling catheters may be used to decrease the risk of urethral trauma associated with indwelling catheters. As reviewed by Feifer and colleagues,[34] early studies evaluating the use of suprapubic catheters "...reported accelerated renal deterioration and lower urinary tract complications, including stones, recurrent infections and blocked catheters. Procedural complications were generally rare. In contrast, recent investigations, in which patients were managed with anticholinergic medications, frequent catheter changes and bladder washing, and volume maintenance procedures demonstrated similar morbidity profiles to CIC.[34]"

Silver-coated and antibiotic-coated catheters

Recently, new catheters coated with silver or antibiotics have been developed to potentially reduce the CAUTIs. A large multicenter trial[35] evaluating short-term use of antimicrobial catheters in hospitalized adults did not find evidence to support their routine use. Neither silver-coated nor nitrofural-coated catheters produced clinically significant reductions in CAUTI in a randomized trial of hospitalized adults. Numerous others have assessed silver-coated or nitrofurazone-coated catheters, some finding short-term reductions in bacteriuria or CAUTI.[36] However, long-term evidence is lacking.

Bladder irrigation

Irrigation is commonly performed by persons with SCI & D who use chronic indwelling catheters for long-term bladder management. In addition, bladder irrigation with antimicrobial agents is sometimes used for persons on IC. However, current guidelines do not recommend routine use of this practice, because evidence is lacking for reduction in CAUTI,[5] and the practice of irrigation may itself increase the risk of CAUTI. No difference in effectiveness has been found between saline and other irrigants, including antibiotic solutions, at reducing bacteriuria.[37] Irrigation solutions in general are not believed to be effective in eliminating bacteriuria.[38]

Fluid Restriction

Fluid management for persons with neurogenic bladder dysfunction can be a challenge. Fluid restrictions of 2 L per day are often used for persons using IC. In addition, persons may need to restrict fluid intake before bedtime. Many persons need to catheterize 1 or more times during the night, especially if a significant postural diuresis occurs. Complicating fluid management further is the dry mouth that may occur with antimuscarinic medications used routinely to improve urine storage capacity. There are no studies specifically evaluating optimal fluid intake in persons with SCI & D.

MEDICAL STRATEGIES FOR UTI PREVENTION AFTER SCI & D

Medical strategies for the prevention of UTIs in individuals with SCI & D have been largely unsuccessful. Therefore, identification of novel agents that can successfully reduce rates of UTIs in individuals with SCI & D is a critical clinical and research objective. The following section reviews the evidence for UTI prevention when using these strategies.

Antibiotic Prophylaxis

Antibiotics are not indicated unless signs or symptoms of illness are present. Signs of systemic illness or sepsis are obvious indications for treatment. Other signs such as changes in the degree of spasticity may or may not indicate a need for antimicrobial therapy. Furthermore, improvement of symptoms after antibiotic treatment does not necessarily correlate with permanent eradication of the infecting organism. Reid[39] reported persistence of antibody labeled bacteria in the bladders of persons with SCI & D on antibiotic therapy.

Use of antibiotic prophylaxis, which is often successful in individuals without neurogenic bladder dysfunction, is less effective in the population with SCI & D. This situation may be because of rapid recolonization and development of bacterial resistance. In addition, non–antibiotic-based medical therapies, including methenamine salts (mandelate or hippurate), have also been unsuccessful. Individuals with SCI & D who use urinary catheters have high rates of bacterial colonization that occur within

30 days of initial catheterization and return to baseline levels after discontinuation of antibiotic therapy.[1] Therefore, follow-up urine cultures are usually unhelpful.

Nonantibiotic Prophylaxis

A multitude of over-the-counter and prescription products exist for prevention or treatment of UTIs (**Table 2**). Many of these products are poorly studied, studied in limited populations, or have been studied with mostly negative or conflicting results. The wide variety of agents attests to the scope of UTIs as a public health problem.

Cranberry

Cranberry products have been shown to reduce the ability of bacteria to adhere to the urinary tract walls. Results with standard cranberry preparations have been mixed. In the largest study to date, Lee and colleagues[40] found no benefit of oral cranberry capsules, methenamine hippurate, or the combination in preventing UTIs. Because of a lack of evidence to support the addition of urinary acidification, it was not used in the study. Hess and colleagues[41] reported benefits in reduction of UTI in 47 patients with SCI & D for any given month while on cranberry over a 6-month period. However, almost 75% of this group used external/condom catheters as their primary method of bladder drainage, making results difficult to interpret. Linsenmeyer and colleagues,[42] in a 4-week study, found no difference in bacteria or leukocyte counts for patients with SCI & D randomized to cranberry supplementation compared with placebo.

Table 2
Nonantibiotic agents used for prevention of bladder infection

Agent	Level I Evidence?
Ascorbic acid	No
Cranberry compounds (*Vaccinium macrocarpon*)	Yes (1b)
Concentrated proanthocyanidins (ellura [Trophikos, LLC Atlanta, GA])	Yes (1b)
Cran-Actin (ascorbic acid, D-mannose, cranberry) (Solaray, Neutraceutical International Corp, Park City, UT)	No
D-Mannose	Yes (1b)
Hyophen (Star Pharmaceuticals, Stellar Biopharma, East Brunswick, NJ)[a,b]	No
Methenamine hippurate/mandelate	No
Methylene blue	No
Herbals	No
Green tea extract (*Camellia sinensis*)	No
Probiotics	No
Lactobacillus spp	No
Bacterial interference	Yes (1b)
Nonpathogenic *Escherichia coli*	Yes (1b)
OM-89 (immunostimulant)	Yes (1b)
Intravesical irrigation/installation	No
Heparin, gentamicin, neomycin, acetic acid, saline	No

[a] Contains: methenamine hippurate, benzoic acid, phenyl salicylate, methylene blue, hyoscyamine sulfate.
[b] Also known as: Atrosept, Cystemms-V, Darcalma, Darpaz, Dolsed, Hyophen, MHP-A, MSP-Blu, Phosenamine, Phosphasal, Prosed DS, Prosed EC, Trac Tabs 2x, UR N-C, Urapine, Urelle, Uretron, Uretron DS, Uribel, Urimar-T, Urimax, Urin D/S, Urised, UriSym, Uritact DS, Uritact-EC, Uritin, Uro Blue, Usept, Ustell, Uta, UTICAP, Utira, Utira-C, Utrona, Utrona-C.

Jepson and Craig, in a Cochrane review published in 2008, reported that "there is some evidence that cranberry juice may decrease the number of symptomatic UTIs over a 12 month period, particularly for women with recurrent UTIs. Its effectiveness for other groups was less certain. The large number of dropouts/withdrawals indicates that cranberry juice may not be acceptable as a long-term treatment option. However, properly designed studies with relevant outcomes are needed.[43]" The investigators concluded that cranberry products cannot be recommended for prevention of recurrent UTIs. More recently, a cranberry supplement with a higher concentration of the presumed active ingredient, proanthocyanidins, has shown efficacy in women.[44] Studies in SCI & D have not been completed, but we are currently conducting a clinical trial evaluating the effects of a standard-dose proanthocyanidin compound, available as an oral supplement called ellura (Trophikos, LLC Atlanta, GA), on both bacteriuria and pyuria in the SCI & D population.

The in vitro effects of cranberry proanthocyanidins in the prevention of adhesion by P-fimbriated uropathogenic *Escherichia coli* are well described. Specifically, a dose-response relationship between proanthocyanidins and a decrease in bacterial virulence has been established.[45,46] However, only a few in vivo trials have examined the use of cranberry ingredients to reduce the recurrence of UTIs in patients in the general population over an extended period.[44,47,48] Comparisons are difficult to make because of the lack of characterization of the supplements used and nonstandardized amount of proanthocyanidins present in the treatments.

D-Mannose

Products containing D-mannose alone or in combination with cranberry based compounds (eg, Cran-Actin [Solaray, Neutraceutical International Corp, Park City, UT]) are in frequent use. Kranjcec and colleagues found a lower risk of recurrent UTIs in women taking D-mannose powder (15%) or nitrofurantoin (20%) versus no prophylaxis (60%) during a 6-month period.[49,50] In addition, the D-mannose group had significantly fewer side effects. Women with interstitial cystitis, diabetes, urinary tract anomalies, or those taking hormone therapy were excluded. We found no studies of D-mannose specifically in persons with SCI & D.

Methenamine

Kevorkian and colleagues[51] found a lower occurrence of UTI in a small group of persons with SCI & D taking methenamine plus urinary acidification with ammonium chloride versus no treatment. As mentioned earlier, Lee and colleagues[40] found no effect of methenamine alone. There are also a variety of prescription products containing methenamine mandelate or hippurate combined with methylene blue, salicylates, and urinary acidifiers (benzoic acid) or pH buffers (sodium phosphate). Whether these cocktail formulations have superior efficacy is not known, because these agents are not well studied. Recent CAUTI guidelines state that methenamine salts should not be used routinely for prevention, but when used, urinary pH should be maintained lower than 6.0.[5]

Bacterial interference

Darouiche and colleagues,[52,53] in 2 separate prospective studies, have found that persons whose bladders were colonized with *E coli* 83972 are significantly less likely to develop a UTI during follow-up. Beereport and colleagues[54] performed a recent review and meta-analysis of randomized controlled trials of nonantibiotic prophylaxis for adults with recurrent UTIs. These investigators evaluated the efficacy, safety, and tolerability of available agents. Seventeen studies met criteria for analysis. The oral immunostimulant OM-89 decreased the rate of UTI recurrence, with a good safety profile. However, there are no specific studies of this agent, which is derived from heat-killed *E coli* serotypes, in persons with neurogenic bladder dysfunction. These investigators' meta-analysis also reported efficacy for cranberry in reducing UTI recurrence in 2 studies.

SUMMARY

There is no broadly applied equipment, medication, or management strategy that has been successful in reducing UTIs to zero or near-zero levels in a population of persons with SCI & D. The incidence of UTIs and recurrent UTIs in persons with SCI & D remains at high levels. Further research and development of nonantimicrobial agents, as well as treatments to normalize function, are important to reduce the impact of this important problem.

REFERENCES

1. Darouiche RO. Infection and spinal cord injury. In: Lin V, editor. Spinal cord medicine: principles and practice. 2nd edition. New York: Demos; 2010. p. 263–9.
2. Siroky MB. Pathogenesis of bacteriuria and infection in the spinal cord injured patient. Am J Med 2002;113(Suppl 1A):67S–79S.
3. Linsenmeyer TA. Neurogenic bladder following spinal cord injury. In: Kirshblum S, Campagnolo DI, editors. Spinal cord medicine. 2nd edition. Philadelphia: Lippincott Williams & Wilkins; 2011. p. 211–41.
4. Singh M, Perkash I, Bodner DR. Urologic management in spinal cord injury. In: Lin V, editor. Spinal cord medicine: principles and practice. 2nd edition. New York: Demos; 2010. p. 362–8.
5. Hooton TM, Bradley SF, Cardenas DD, et al. Diagnosis, prevention, and treatment of catheter-associated urinary tract infection in adults: 2009 International Clinical Practice Guidelines from the Infectious Diseases Society of America. Clin Infect Dis 2010;50(5):625–63.
6. Stover SL, Lloyd LK, Waites KB, et al. Urinary tract infection in spinal cord injury. Arch Phys Med Rehabil 1989;70(1):47–54.
7. Goetz LL, Cardenas DD, Kennelly M, et al. International spinal cord injury urinary tract infection basic data set. Spinal Cord 2013;51(9):700–4.
8. Massa LM, Hoffman JM, Cardenas DD. Validity, accuracy, and predictive value of urinary tract infection signs and symptoms in individuals with spinal cord injury on intermittent catheterization. J Spinal Cord Med 2009;32(5):568–73.
9. Linsenmeyer TA, Oakley A. Accuracy of individuals with spinal cord injury at predicting urinary tract infections based on their symptoms. J Spinal Cord Med 2003;26(4):352–7.
10. The prevention and management of urinary tract infections among people with spinal cord injuries. National Institute on Disability and Rehabilitation Research consensus statement. January 27-29, 1992. J Am Paraplegia Soc 1992;15(3):194–204.
11. Biering-Sorensen F, Charlifue S, DeVivo M, et al. International spinal cord injury data sets. Spinal Cord 2006;44(9):530–4.
12. Biering-Sorensen F, Craggs M, Kennelly M, et al. International lower urinary tract function basic spinal cord injury data set. Spinal Cord 2008;46(5):325–30.
13. Biering-Sorensen F, Craggs M, Kennelly M, et al. International urodynamic basic spinal cord injury data set. Spinal Cord 2008;46(7):513–6.
14. Biering-Sorensen F, Craggs M, Kennelly M, et al. International urinary tract imaging basic spinal cord injury data set. Spinal Cord 2009;47(5):379–83.

15. Biering-Sorensen F, Charlifue S, Devivo MJ, et al. Incorporation of the international spinal cord injury data set elements into the National Institute of Neurological Disorders and Stroke common data elements. Spinal Cord 2011;49(1):60–4.

16. Klausner AP, Steers WD. The neurogenic bladder: an update with management strategies for primary care physicians. Med Clin North Am 2011;95(1):111–20.

17. Wein AJ. Classification of neurogenic voiding dysfunction. J Urol 1981;125(5): 605–9.

18. Wein AJ. Lower urinary tract dysfunction in neurologic injury and disease. In: Wein AJ, Kavoussi LR, Novick AC, et al, editors. Campbell-Walsh urology. Philadelphia: Saunders Elsevier; 2007. p. 2011–45, 8.

19. Hackler RH, Hall MK, Zampieri TA. Bladder hypocompliance in the spinal cord injury population. J Urol 1989;141(6):1390–3.

20. Weld KJ, Graney MJ, Dmochowski RR. Differences in bladder compliance with time and associations of bladder management with compliance in spinal cord injured patients. J Urol 2000;163(4):1228–33.

21. McGuire EJ, Woodside JR, Borden TA, et al. Prognostic value of urodynamic testing in myelodysplastic patients. J Urol 1981;126(2):205–9.

22. Edokpolo LU, Stavris KB, Foster HE Jr. Intermittent catheterization and recurrent urinary tract infection in spinal cord injury. Top Spinal Cord Inj Rehabil 2012; 18(2):187–92.

23. Consortium for Spinal Cord Medicine. Bladder management following spinal cord injury: what you should know. A guide for people with spinal cord injury. Washington, DC: Paralyzed Veterans of America; 2010.

24. Hudson E, Murahata RI. The 'no-touch' method of intermittent urinary catheter insertion: can it reduce the risk of bacteria entering the bladder? Spinal Cord 2005;43(10):611–4.

25. Giannantoni A, Di Stasi SM, Scivoletto G, et al. Intermittent catheterization with a prelubricated catheter in spinal cord injured patients: a prospective randomized crossover study. J Urol 2001;166(1):130–3.

26. Bennett CJ, Young MN, Razi SS, et al. The effect of urethral introducer tip catheters on the incidence of urinary tract infection outcomes in spinal cord injured patients. J Urol 1997;158(2):519–21.

27. De Ridder DJ, Everaert K, Fernandez LG, et al. Intermittent catheterisation with hydrophilic-coated catheters (SpeediCath) reduces the risk of clinical urinary tract infection in spinal cord injured patients: a prospective randomised parallel comparative trial. Eur Urol 2005;48(6):991–5.

28. Stensballe J, Looms D, Nielsen PN, et al. Hydrophilic-coated catheters for intermittent catheterisation reduce urethral micro trauma: a prospective, randomised, participant-blinded, crossover study of three different types of catheters. Eur Urol 2005;48(6):978–83.

29. Cardenas DD, Hoffman JM. Hydrophilic catheters versus noncoated catheters for reducing the incidence of urinary tract infections: a randomized controlled trial. Arch Phys Med Rehabil 2009;90(10):1668–71.

30. Cardenas DD, Moore KN, Dannels-McClure A, et al. Intermittent catheterization with a hydrophilic-coated catheter delays urinary tract infections in acute spinal cord injury: a prospective, randomized, multicenter trial. PM R 2011;3(5):408–17.

31. Cardenas DD, Hooton TM. Urinary tract infection in persons with spinal cord injury. Arch Phys Med Rehabil 1995;76(3):272–80.

32. Yang CC, Mayo ME. External urethral sphincterotomy: long-term follow-up. Neurourol Urodyn 1995;14(1):25–31.

33. Kim YH, Bird ET, Priebe M, et al. The role of oxybutynin in spinal cord injured patients with indwelling catheters. J Urol 1997;158(6):2083–6.
34. Feifer A, Corcos J. Contemporary role of suprapubic cystostomy in treatment of neuropathic bladder dysfunction in spinal cord injured patients. Neurourol Urodyn 2008;27(6):475–9.
35. Pickard R, Lam T, MacLennan G, et al. Antimicrobial catheters for reduction of symptomatic urinary tract infection in adults requiring short-term catheterisation in hospital: a multicentre randomised controlled trial. Lancet 2012;380(9857): 1927–35.
36. Al Mohajer M, Darouiche RO. Prevention and treatment of urinary catheter-associated infections. Curr Infect Dis Rep 2013;15(2):116–23.
37. Waites KB, Canupp KC, Roper JF, et al. Evaluation of 3 methods of bladder irrigation to treat bacteriuria in persons with neurogenic bladder. J Spinal Cord Med 2006;29(3):217–26.
38. Cravens DD, Zweig S. Urinary catheter management. Am Fam Physician 2000; 61(2):369–76.
39. Reid G. Do antibiotics clear bladder infections? J Urol 1994;152(3):865–7.
40. Lee BB, Haran MJ, Hunt LM, et al. Spinal-injured neuropathic bladder antisepsis (SINBA) trial. Spinal Cord 2007;45(8):542–50.
41. Hess MJ, Hess PE, Sullivan MR, et al. Evaluation of cranberry tablets for the prevention of urinary tract infections in spinal cord injured patients with neurogenic bladder. Spinal Cord 2008;46(9):622–6.
42. Linsenmeyer TA, Harrison B, Oakley A, et al. Evaluation of cranberry supplement for reduction of urinary tract infections in individuals with neurogenic bladders secondary to spinal cord injury. A prospective, double-blinded, placebo-controlled, crossover study. J Spinal Cord Med 2004;27(1):29–34.
43. Jepson RG, Craig JC. Cranberries for preventing urinary tract infections. Cochrane Database Syst Rev 2008;(1):CD001321.
44. Beerepoot MA, ter Riet G, Nys S, et al. Cranberries vs antibiotics to prevent urinary tract infections: a randomized double-blind noninferiority trial in premenopausal women. Arch Intern Med 2011;171(14):1270–8.
45. Howell AB, Botto H, Combescure C, et al. Dosage effect on uropathogenic *Escherichia coli* anti-adhesion activity in urine following consumption of cranberry powder standardized for proanthocyanidin content: a multicentric randomized double blind study. BMC Infect Dis 2010;10:94.
46. Lavigne JP, Bourg G, Combescure C, et al. In-vitro and in-vivo evidence of dose-dependent decrease of uropathogenic *Escherichia coli* virulence after consumption of commercial *Vaccinium macrocarpon* (cranberry) capsules. Clin Microbiol Infect 2008;14(4):350–5.
47. Stothers L. A randomized trial to evaluate effectiveness and cost effectiveness of naturopathic cranberry products as prophylaxis against urinary tract infection in women. Can J Urol 2002;9(3):1558–62.
48. Wing DA, Rumney PJ, Preslicka CW, et al. Daily cranberry juice for the prevention of asymptomatic bacteriuria in pregnancy: a randomized, controlled pilot study. J Urol 2008;180(4):1367–72.
49. Kranjcec B, Papes D, Altarac S. D-mannose powder for prophylaxis of recurrent urinary tract infections in women: a randomized clinical trial. World J Urol 2014; 32(1):79–84.
50. Altarac S, Papes D. Use of D-mannose in prophylaxis of recurrent urinary tract infections (UTIs) in women. BJU Int 2014;113(1):9–10.

51. Kevorkian CG, Merritt JL, Ilstrup DM. Methenamine mandelate with acidification: an effective urinary antiseptic in patients with neurogenic bladder. Mayo Clin Proc 1984;59(8):523–9.

52. Darouiche RO, Green BG, Donovan WH, et al. Multicenter randomized controlled trial of bacterial interference for prevention of urinary tract infection in patients with neurogenic bladder. Urology 2011;78(2):341–6.

53. Darouiche RO, Thornby JI, Cerra-Stewart C, et al. Bacterial interference for prevention of urinary tract infection: a prospective, randomized, placebo-controlled, double-blind pilot trial. Clin Infect Dis 2005;41(10):1531–4.

54. Beerepoot MA, Geerlings SE, van Haarst EP, et al. Nonantibiotic prophylaxis for recurrent urinary tract infections: a systematic review and meta-analysis of randomized controlled trials. J Urol 2013;190(6):1981–9.

Diaphragmatic Pacing in Spinal Cord Injury

Kevin Dalal, MD[a],*, Anthony F. DiMarco, MD[b]

KEYWORDS

- Diaphragm • Phrenic nerve • Tetraplegia

KEY POINTS

- The diaphragm is innervated by cervical nerves C3 to C5, but a patient may be able to mobilize the diaphragm with only partial innervation of the diaphragm.
- Testing diaphragm function may be accomplished with the "sniff test" of diaphragm elevation under fluoroscopy. Further, electrodiagnostic testing of phrenic nerve function also may be used to show a response in diaphragm function.
- Diaphragm pacing has been shown to be an effective way of weaning and maintaining patients off of mechanical ventilation, thus lowering the care burden, and liberating the patient to be more mobile, and lessening the potential for morbidity.

INTRODUCTION

There are more than 11,000 new cases of spinal cord injury (SCI) each year. Approximately 50% of these patients have tetraplegia, and of those, approximately 4% require mechanical ventilation long term.[1] The patient with tetraplegia faces significant challenges beyond the mobility and sensory impairments imposed by the injury. Chief among these issues is that of respiratory impairment. Patients with tetraplegia, depending on whether the injury is complete or incomplete, will have varying degrees of respiratory dysfunction based on the amount of residually intact innervation to the muscles of inspiration and expiration. The muscles of expiration include the abdominal musculature and intercostals, which are innervated by nerves coming from the thoracic cord, and are less likely to be functionally intact in a patient with a cervical injury. The chief muscle of inspiration is the diaphragm, which is innervated by motoneurons from the cervical spinal cord, and thus susceptible to dysfunction in tetraplegia.

The standard of care for patients who cannot adequately mobilize their diaphragm (in addition to a host of other comorbidities that could compromise respiratory

Disclosure: The author has no financial disclosures.
a Department of Physical Medicine and Rehabilitation, University of Miami-Miller School of Medicine, 1120 North West 14th Street, Suite 936, Miami, FL 33136, USA; b Rammelkamp Research Center, MetroHealth Medical Center, 2500 MetroHealth Drive, Cleveland, OH 44109, USA
* Corresponding author.
E-mail address: kdalal@med.miami.edu

Phys Med Rehabil Clin N Am 25 (2014) 619–629
http://dx.doi.org/10.1016/j.pmr.2014.04.004
1047-9651/14/$ – see front matter © 2014 Elsevier Inc. All rights reserved.

function) is to perform a tracheostomy and mechanically ventilate the patient. This article outlines the negative implications of mechanical ventilation, and discusses the possibility and benefits of allowing the patient to breathe with the assistance of exogenous diaphragm pacing.

PHYSIOLOGY OF BREATHING

As previously mentioned, the primary muscle of inspiration is the diaphragm, a thin, dome-shaped sheet of skeletal muscle, with muscular tissue converging on a central tendon that forms the crest of the dome. The muscle fibers originate from various structures, including the lumbar vertebrae and abdominal wall posteriorly, the ribs laterally, and the xiphoid process and floating ribs anteriorly. The central tendon is closer to the anterior of the thorax and, thus, the posterior muscle fibers are longer, traveling a farther course to converge on the tendon. The diaphragm is pierced by 3 apertures, which allow passage of the vena cava, the esophagus, and the aorta.[2]

During inspiration, the diaphragm contracts, which creates a negative-pressure vacuum, and draws air into the thoracic cavity through the respiratory system. The diaphragm contracts volitionally during the daytime hours and automatically during sleep, based on CO_2 levels monitored in the brain's respiratory centers. When the diaphragm relaxes, air is exhaled by the elastic recoil of the lung and the pleural cavity. In forced exhalation, such as a cough, the internal intercostal muscles and abdominal muscles work antagonistically to the diaphragm. Additionally, the diaphragm can be used in nonrespiratory capacities by suddenly increasing intra-abdominal pressure, as in the processes of vomiting, defecating, and urination.

The diaphragm is innervated by the phrenic motoneurons, which are supplied by cervical spinal nerves C3, C4, and C5. These spinal nerves combine peripherally to form the paired phrenic nerves, which progress caudally through the thorax and insert into the diaphragm. In the event of a cervical SCI, the interruption of respiratory bulbospinal pathways can lead to respiratory paresis or paralysis.

In higher-level cervical injuries, the spinal roots, which directly contribute to the phrenic nerves and innervate the diaphragm, are spared, but the roots from the respiratory centers in the medulla to the cord are still interrupted. These patients will definitely require exogenous ventilation. However, there are many disadvantages to mechanical ventilation, and these higher-level injuries may be candidates for diaphragm pacing.

MECHANICAL VENTILATION

In such cases of acute or chronic respiratory failure, the use of positive-pressure mechanical ventilation can serve as a life-sustaining measure. Some patients may tolerate less-invasive means of mechanical ventilation, but at least initially, many patients are managed via the traditional measure of positive-pressure ventilation via a tracheostomy.[3] Up to 20% of newly injured patients with SCI may require mechanical ventilation initially, but many patients improve in the following weeks. Regardless, between 200 and 400 patients per year become dependent on lifelong ventilator support.[4]

However, mechanical ventilation is susceptible to increased morbidity from pneumonia, as well as earlier mortality.[5] When compared with an able-bodied 20-year-old, the life expectancy for a 20-year-old patient with SCI on long-term mechanical ventilation decreases markedly from 58.6 to only 17.1 years. According to the National Spinal Cord Injury 2002 Database, survival rates decreased from 84% in the nonventilated patient to only 33% in the ventilated population.[1]

Unfortunately, mechanical ventilation presents several obstacles for the patient, especially in light of the compounded impact on independence and mobility beyond that imposed by the injury's impact on motor function in the extremities. Additionally, mechanical ventilation imposes varying degrees of physical discomfort, and impairments in speech and olfaction.[6] The cost and care burden of total mechanical ventilation can make living in the home environment impossible, thus shifting more of the care responsibilities to long-term facilities. Care of a ventilated patient may cost up to $200,000 per year, and lifetime costs are outlined in **Table 1**.[7] The care of the ventilated patient requires 24-hour supervision by a trained caregiver. The caregiver must feel comfortable in manipulating ventilator settings to optimize the respiratory function and adapt to periodic changes in oxygenation. Also, the caregiver must be able to provide adequate pulmonary toilet, whether it is via chest percussion to loosen secretions or provide frequent suctioning.[8]

PHRENIC NERVE PACING

In patients with respiratory failure secondary to a cervical SCI, mechanical ventilation is a lifesaving intervention. Under certain circumstances, some patients may be able to wean to noninvasive ventilation or use noninvasive ventilation for short periods of time. More typically, patients are subjected to positive-pressure ventilation with a tracheostomy. However, the use of mechanical ventilation impairs speech and olfaction, and leads to atrophy of the diaphragm muscle fibers.[8]

The advantages of avoiding ventilation include reduction in airway pressure, increased posterior lobe ventilation, and maintenance of negative chest pressures.[8] Phrenic nerve pacing is a more realistic approximation of the patient's native respiratory drive in that it proceeds via negative-pressure ventilation by contraction of the patient's own muscle fibers as opposed to exogenously induced inflation. Speech quality is improved with the lessened noise, better enabling the voice to be heard. Olfaction is improved, which in turn improves the patient's sense of well-being.[6] Phrenic nerve pacing also has more cosmesis when compared with the extensive tubing, machinery, and noise associated with a mechanical ventilator. Shedding the tethering to this ancillary machinery also obviously liberates the patient for increased household and community mobility and hence may lead to increased reintegration into society.

DIRECT DIAPHRAGM PACING

Exogenous electrical stimulation of the phrenic nerve has been a viable treatment option, given appropriate physiologic circumstances, for more than 30 years. Until

Table 1				
Costs related to ventilator dependancy in spinal cord injury				
Severity of Injury	Average Yearly Expenses 1st Year	Average Yearly Expenses Subsequent	Estimated Lifetime Costs 25 y old	Estimated Lifetime Cost 50 y old
High (C1–C4) Tetraplegia	$775,567	$139,923	$3,059,184	$1,800,958
Low (C5–C8) Tetraplegia	$500,829	$56,905	$1,729,754	$1,095,411

From National Spinal Cord Injury Statistical Center, Birmingham, AL – January 2008; and McCrory DC, Samsa GP, Hamilton GG, et al. Treatment of pulmonary disease following cervical spinal cord injury: evidence reports/technology assessments, no. 27. Rockville (MD): Agency for Healthcare Research and Quality (US); 2001.

recently, direct electrical stimulation of the phrenic nerves was the standard procedure for this kind of intervention, but required a thoracotomy or neck surgery for electrode placement and the surgical manipulation posed a risk of damaging the nerves themselves. A less-invasive procedure allowing percutaneous placement of electrodes over strategically located areas of the diaphragm has emerged as a viable alternative with reduced risk. As far back as 1980, Mortimer demonstrated that the diaphragm could be directly stimulated at its motor points. The motor points are determined using laparoscopy via electrical stimulation on the abdominal surface of the diaphragm.[8]

SELECTION CRITERIA

The placement of a diaphragm pacemaker comes with very specific criteria for selecting potential surgical candidates. The grade and level of injury is of paramount importance. An injury at any level can theoretically tolerate mechanical ventilation, but patients with C3-level to C5-level injuries cannot be paced because of the Wallerian degeneration that affects the phrenic nerves and, thus, would not respond to pacing. In such patients, diaphragmatic pacing is not an option because the motor pools and phrenic nerves are not intact. One criterion for placement is that the lesion must typically be above the third cervical level. The cell bodies of the nerves that supply the phrenic nerve are C3 to C5 and must be intact for the diaphragm or phrenic nerve to be paced.

Patients who are candidates for phrenic nerve or diaphragmatic pacing are almost universally on mechanical ventilation at the time of that determination. The assessment of the patient's ventilatory status and the viability of the phrenic nerves are the primary determinants of candidacy for pacing. A patient cannot sustain spontaneous breathing with a vital capacity less than 10 mL/kg and a maximum inspiratory pressure of less than 20 cm H20.

There also remain certain physiologic limitations when compared with normal physiologic breathing. First and most obviously, as the breathing mechanism is now being exogenously paced, there is no spontaneous control of breathing. Important to consider, as well, is that only the inspiratory aspect of the breathing mechanism is facilitated by pacing the diaphragm. The muscles of expiration are not stimulated, which means the patient's cough mechanism will continue to be greatly impaired. This will leave the patient susceptible to having difficulty clearing secretions, and thus prone to atelectasis and pneumonia.

ELECTRODIAGNOSTIC TESTING

Phrenic motor nerve conduction studies (NCSs) are used in the preoperative evaluation of diaphragmatic pacing candidates. Damage to the anterior horn cells and the phrenic nerve axons result in a decrease in the diaphragm's compound muscle action potential (CMAP), as well as abnormalities in the motor unit action potential and fibrillation potentials.[9] For a patient to be considered a candidate for pacing, active phrenic nerve function must be established. To determine diaphragm viability, there should be a recordable CMAP response using NCSs, preferably in conjunction with movement under fluoroscopy.[10]

The diaphragm's inferior movement on phrenic nerve stimulation can be visualized via fluoroscopy for a more reliable, less operator-dependent evaluation of phrenic nerve function. The diaphragm should be expected to descend at least 3 to 4 cm on cervical phrenic nerve stimulation.[11] These findings should be correlated with other objective measures of diaphragm function, such as the sniff test, which is fluoroscopic measurement of diaphragm movement during rapid inhalation.

Initially, a more transient conduction block may be caused by edema or other trauma-related anatomic distortions. Such conditions may resolve quickly and manifest more rapidly improving CMAP responses than those predicted in cases requiring actual axonal regeneration.

Each phrenic nerve in question is stimulated in the neck approximating the sternocleidomastoid and placing the bipolar stimulator in the supraclavicular fossa between the sternal and clavicular heads of the sternocleidomastoid muscle, with the patient lying supine.[10] The active recording electrode is placed on the sternum above the xiphoid process and the reference electrode is placed on the lower costal margin along the anterior axillary line. The current intensity is increased to obtain a supramaximal CMAP (20% greater than required for maximal CMAP). Multiple stimulations are helpful to confirm reproducibility. Also, repositioning of the stimulator may be helpful in preventing costimulation of ipsilateral chest wall muscles innervated by the brachial plexus (**Fig. 1**).[10]

Improvements in CMAP amplitudes over time were positive prognosticators for improvement in diaphragm function. Serial testing of the phrenic nerve may be performed for up to 2 years after SCI to track potential improvement despite small initial CMAP responses.[9]

WEANING FROM MECHANICAL VENTILATION

Most patients who will be placed on diaphragm pacing will be doing so in the setting of mechanical ventilation. This switch from one modality to another must be performed carefully to optimize the transition process. In mechanical ventilation, there is baseline hyperventilation and low bicarbonate stores secondary to reduced partial pressure of carbon dioxide. Because pacing invokes a more natural ventilatory physiology, the patient may feel dyspneic although ventilation is appropriate. To facilitate the acclimation to the transition, it is advisable to reduce the respiratory rate and volume for a period of several days before the switch. This will help prevent any inevitable acidosis.

One other key component of the transition process is the conditioning of the diaphragm. Because many patients who are selected for pacer placement may have been on mechanical ventilation for many months if not years, the disuse atrophy that

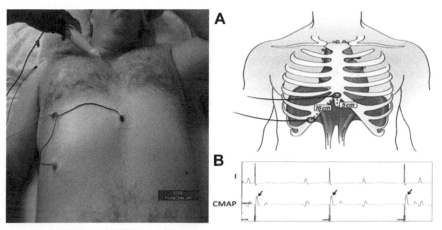

Fig. 1. Phrenic nerve conduction study technique. (*A*) Photo and diagram: Phrenic nerve stimulated in supraclavicular fossa. Active recording electrode on sternum and reference electrode on lower costal margin. (*B*) Supramaximal CMAP reading.

has occurred benefits from a graded, stepwise reversal process. The practitioner can elect to increase pacing periods as a proportion of each hour (5, then 10, then 15 minutes) and increasing these intervals to the next interval on a week-to-week basis.

The initiation of pacing intervals and their subsequent increases typically are performed during the waking hours initially. The patient is allowed to "rest" at night on mechanical ventilation. Once the pacing intervals are increased to the point that the patient is being paced full time during waking hours, the intervals can begin during the sleeping hours.

EQUIPMENT

Direct electrical stimulation to the phrenic nerve requires a thoracotomy and physical manipulation of the phrenic nerves, which incurs more morbidity. However, intramuscular diaphragm pacing has the advantage of requiring only minimally invasive laparoscopy.

Avery Laboratories (Commack, NY) was the first company to start providing equipment for pacing, as they have been doing so for nearly 30 years. Using this equipment requires surgical incisions with direct stimulation of the phrenic nerve. More recently, Synapse Biomedical (Oberlin, OH), with its NeuRx system, has been approved by the Food and Drug Administration for use. The NeuRx system is a less-invasive, external pulse generator that provides percutaneous pacing of the diaphragm.

The equipment involved includes radiofrequency receivers and electrodes (4) that are surgically implanted on the abdominal surface of the diaphragm. The external components include a stimulus transmitter, antennae, and a battery source, which is connected directly to the electrodes. Diaphragm pacing incurs higher initial costs and a surgical procedure for implantation when compared with mechanical ventilation. However, longitudinally, the costs are amortized over time without the need for the upkeep and maintenance of mechanical ventilation. However, a backup mechanical ventilation system has to be in place in case of equipment failure. At the very least, an Ambu bag for manual ventilation must be on hand if necessary.

NORMAL PHYSIOLOGY

In spontaneous, normal breathing, the respiratory center of the medulla generates the respiratory drive and dictates the rate and volume of respiration. This signal can be affected by higher centers in the brain, as well as central and peripheral chemoreceptors in the lungs and chest wall.[3] Inspiration involves a coordinated contraction of multiple muscles, namely the diaphragm, intercostals, and accessory muscles, and results in negative intrathoracic pressure, which draws air into the lungs. Expiration, on the other hand is a passive process.

The individual motor units are classified into 4 subtypes: Type I, Type IIa, Type IIx, and Type IIb. Their characteristics are summarized in **Table 2**.[12]

Table 2 Muscle fiber types			
Type	Speed	Fatigability	Oxidative
Type I	Slow twitch	Resistant	Highly oxidative
Type IIa	Fast twitch	Resistant	Highly oxidative
Type IIx	Fast twitch	Intermediate	
Type IIb	Fast twitch	Fatigable	Glycolytic

In the course of normal, healthy respiration, the diaphragm is under constant demand. This demand is enabled by a proportionately high number of fatigue-resistant fibers, as well as a recruitment pattern that favors small, slow units initially, and the progressive recruitment of the more fatigable fast fibers that generate greater forces.[3]

The diaphragm is innervated by motor neurons at the C3, 4, and 5 spinal levels. A C4-level or C5-level SCI would therefore compromise the anterior horn cells and accompanying rootlets that supply the axons to the phrenic nerve.

PHYSIOLOGY OF VENTILATION

The impact of exogenously imposing ventilation through the respiratory apparatus can have a long-standing negative impact on the patient. The patient's native musculature is not being stimulated, but rather artificially inflated. A study in the New England Journal of Medicine compared biopsy samples from the diaphragms of 14 brain-dead organ donor controls with 8 patient control subjects who did not have mechanical ventilation.[13] The case subjects were subjected to mechanical ventilation for between 18 and 69 hours. After just 18 hours of positive-pressure ventilation, there was marked atrophy noted in the diaphragm fibers, with a 57% decrease in Type 1 slow-twitch fibers and a 53% decrease in fast-twitch fibers. The active muscle areas atrophy faster, which downstream leads to oxidative stress and increased proteolysis.[13]

PHYSIOLOGY OF PACING

In contrast, phrenic or diaphragm pacing induces phenotypic changes to the patient's native anatomy, which alters the physiology of respiratory function when compared with uninjured cohorts. Diaphragms subjected to pacing experience the stimulation effects most acutely on the largest-diameter axons, which represents a reversal of the recruitment order previously discussed. Also, chronic phrenic nerve pacing will, over time, shift the proportion of Type I and II fibers from being equally distributed to being more uniformly Type I.[14]

MORBIDITY AND MORTALITY

Although the systems have greatly improved over time, with any foreign body requiring surgical intervention, there are associated risks, especially considering the vulnerabilities of this patient population. Such failures typically include battery or receiver failure and breakage of antenna wires. Systems typically have low-battery alarms to prevent such events from arising. As with any implantation of foreign bodies, there is an associated risk of infection, albeit relatively minor.

One potential physiologic complication comes with the use of pacing in a younger patient. Because of high lung compliance in patients younger than 15, there is a paradoxic inward movement of the chest wall with negative-pressure ventilation, which effectively reduces the inspired volume. As compliance decreases after the age of 15 and with prolonged time from SCI as well, this effect tends to stabilize.[15]

EXPIRATORY MUSCLE FUNCTION

Unlike the diaphragm, the major expiratory muscles are innervated by several pairs of thoracic nerves. Restoration of expiratory muscle function by stimulation of individual nerve roots therefore is not practical. The expiratory muscles, however, can be electrically activated by stimulation of disc electrodes applied to the dorsal surface of the upper thoracic spinal cord at the T9, T11, and L1 levels (**Fig. 2**). In a pilot study of individuals with cervical or high thoracic SCI, spinal cord stimulation (SCS)

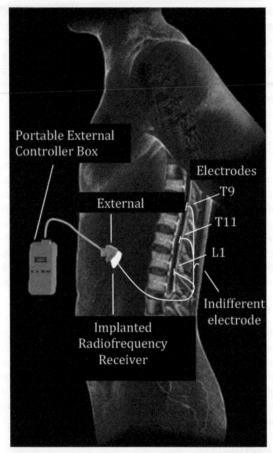

Fig. 2. Electrical stimulation system for cough assist. (*From* DiMarco AF, Kowalski KE, Geertman RT, et al. Lower thoracic spinal cord stimulation to restore cough in patients with spinal cord injury: results of a National Institutes of Health-sponsored clinical trial. Part I: methodology and effectiveness of expiratory muscle activation. Arch Phys Med Rehabil 2009;90:718; with permission.)

of any 2 spinal cord levels in combination has been shown to effectively activate the major bulk of the expiratory muscles resulting in the generation of large positive airway pressures and peak airflow characteristic of an effective cough.[16]

Subjects were trained to activate their expiratory muscles in sequence with the other components of a normal cough reflex (ie, subjects inspired deeply, closed their glottis, and then activated their expiratory muscles, followed by relaxation). As with normal cough, this entire maneuver takes place in less than a second and could be performed on demand. Activation of the expiratory muscles could be achieved by depressing a button on an external control box. The control box could be programmed to provide a multitude of stimulus combinations resulting in various cough intensities and efforts in series (eg, every 10 seconds for 1 to 2 minutes).

Subjects enrolled in the initial clinical trial reported that use of the cough system resulted in significantly greater ease in raising secretions and improvement in life quality.[17] In terms of more objective parameters, there were significant reductions in the need for caregiver support for secretion management and in the incidence of respiratory tract infections at 1-year follow-up. Moreover, long-term follow-up of users for at least 2 years (mean 4.7 years) demonstrated that the individuals continued to use the device on a regular basis and the initial benefits at the 1-year mark were maintained.[18] These suggest that this technique has a high degree of clinical utility with the potential to significantly impact the morbidity and mortality associated with SCI.

Side effects of this technique included leg jerks at high stimulus intensities that were not painful and were well-tolerated. There were also some cases of autonomic dysreflexia (AD) on initial application of stimulation. Signs of AD abated and eventually resolved over several weeks with continued stimulation. There was no incidence of bowel or bladder leakage.

AVAILABILITY

Direct diaphragm pacing (DP) is commercially available by 3 different manufacturers including Avery Laboratories, Atrotech OY (Tampere, Finland), and Medimplant Biotechnisches Labor (Vienna, Austria). Of the 3, only the Avery Laboratories device is available in the United States. Intramuscular DP is commercially available from Synapse Biomedical (Oberlin, OH). On the other hand, the cough system is currently in clinical trials under an Investigational Device Exception with the Food and Drug Administration and not commercially available.

FUTURE DIRECTIONS

Many individuals with SCI are not eligible for DP because of lack of adequate diaphragm function. Preliminary work has demonstrated, however, that intercostal to phrenic nerve transfer may restore phrenic nerve viability and provide many more patients with the option of DP.[19]

With regard to SCS to restore cough, a surgical procedure involving multiple laminotomies is required for electrode placement. A new device using wire electrodes, which can be placed using a minimally invasive technique, is under development. This could be performed on an outpatient as successfully as use of the disc electrodes; this method is likely to improve both physician and subject acceptance of electric stimulation techniques to restore an effective cough.

Although the fundamental concept of electrical stimulation has been known for centuries, and the functional utility of such technology has been available for decades, there have been significant advances in the implementation of this technique in recent years. Initially, direct stimulation of the phrenic nerves themselves required neck surgery and later thoracotomy. Then, advances in technique led to the direct stimulation of the motoneuron areas on each hemidiaphragm. These systems became more practical as the electrodes were attached percutaneously and less invasively. Fully enclosed, implantable systems, analogous to a cardiac pacemaker, will make these systems even easier to use by precluding the risk of loosening connections.

In patients with one disrupted phrenic nerve, pacing of the remaining, stimulatable diaphragm in combination with electric stimulation of intercostal muscles may be used in tandem to optimize function. The upper thoracic nerves that innervate the intercostals are responsible for 35% of inspiratory capacity. A hemilaminectomy must be performed, after which direct stimulation of the upper thoracic ventral roots is accomplished via placement of disc electrodes on the upper thoracic spinal cord.[20] A 2005 study showed that combining hemidiaphragm plus intercostal pacing was superior to either modality alone in terms of volume generation. In a gradual incremental process, a plateau in maximum volume and pressure generation was reached at approximately

10 to 12 weeks. Overall, the efficiency and inspired volume is less than that found in combined bilateral pacing, but it could still serve as a viable option in a patient with one damaged phrenic nerve.[21]

SUMMARY

In the appropriate setting, there are distinct advantages of diaphragm pacing when compared with mechanical ventilation. As discussed, principal among these are the avoidance of the machinery of mechanical ventilation and the associated facility of transport in and out of the home as well as to and from bed. Speech and olfactory sensation are improved. More subtle factors contributing to patient quality of life is the elimination of ventilator noise and tubing. The use of a pacer, even for portions of the day, also helps lessen the burden on caregiver support. Patient anxiety over potential ventilator failure may be ameliorated by using a pacer, but it is important to remember that a backup ventilator system needs to be made available in case of pacer failure. Unfortunately, that means a tracheostomy must be maintained, even if it is not functionally implemented for most of or the entire day. Overall, the physiologic advantage of using the patient's native musculature without the challenges associated with mechanical ventilation will surely lead to improved long-term outcomes.

REFERENCES

1. DeVivo MJ, Go BK, Jackson AB. Overview of the national spinal cord injury statistical center database. J Spinal Cord Med 2002;25:335–8.
2. Drake RL, Vogl AW, Mitchell AWM. Gray's anatomy for students. Toronto, ON: Elsevier/Churchill Livingstone; 2005. p. 134–5.
3. DiMarco AF. Phrenic nerve stimulation in patients with spinal cord injury. Respir Physiolo Neurobiol 2009;169:200–9.
4. Carter RE, Donova WH, Halstead L, et al. Comparative study of electrophrenic nerve stimulation and mechanical ventilator support in traumatic spinal cord injury. Paraplegia 1987;25:86–91.
5. Tedde ML, Filho PV, Hajjar LA, et al. Diaphragmatic pacing stimulation in spinal cord injury: anesthetic and perioperative management. Clinics (Sao Paulo) 2012;67:1265–9.
6. Adler D, Gonzalez-Bermejo J, Duguet A, et al. Diaphragm pacing restores olfaction in tetraplegia. Eur Respir J 2009;34:365–70.
7. Onders RP, Elmo M, Khansarinia S, et al. Complete worldwide operative experience in laparoscopic diaphragm pacing: results and differences in spinal cord injured patients and amyotrophic lateral sclerosis patients. Surg Endosc 2009; 23:1433–40.
8. Jarosz R, Littlepage MM, Creasey G, et al. Functional electrical stimulation in spinal cord injury respiratory care. Top Spinal Cord Inj Rehabil 2012;18:315–21.
9. Strakowski JA, Pease WS, Johnson EW. Phrenic nerve stimulation in the evaluation of ventilator dependent individuals with C4 and C5 level spinal cord injury. Am J Phys Med Rehabil 2007;86:153–7.
10. Alshekhlee A. Phrenic nerve conduction studies in spinal cord injury: applications for diaphragmatic pacing. Muscle Nerve 2008;38:1546–52.
11. DiMarco AF. Diaphragm pacing in patients with spinal cord injury. Top Spinal Cord Inj Rehabil 1999;5(1):6–20.
12. Mantilla CV, Sieck GC. Invited review: mechanisms underlying motor unit plasticity in the respiratory system. J Appl Phys 2003;94:1230–41.

13. Levine S, Nguyen T, Taylor N, et al. Rapid disuse atrophy of diaphragm fibers in mechanically ventilated humans. N Engl J Med 2008;358:1327–35.
14. Glenn WW, Hogan JF, Logan JS, et al. Ventilator support by pacing of the conditioned diaphragm in quadriplegia. N Engl J Med 1984;310(18):1150–5.
15. Weese-Mayer DE, Morrow AS, Brouillette RT, et al. Diaphragm pacing in infants and children. J Pediatr 1992;120:1–8.
16. DiMarco AF, Kowalski KE, Geertman RT, et al. Lower thoracic spinal cord stimulation to restore cough in patients with spinal cord injury: results of a National Institutes of Health-sponsored clinical trial. Part I: methodology and effectiveness of expiratory muscle activation. Arch Phys Med Rehabil 2009;90:717–25.
17. DiMarco AF, Kowalski KE, Geertman RT, et al. Lower thoracic spinal cord stimulation to restore cough in patients with spinal cord injury: results of a National Institutes of Health-sponsored clinical trial. Part II: clinical outcomes. Arch Phys Med Rehabil 2009;90:726–32.
18. DiMarco AF, Kowalski KE, Hromyak DR, et al. Long-term follow-up of spinal cord stimulation (SCS) to restore cough in subjects with spinal cord injury. J Spinal Cord Med 2013. [E-pub ahead of print].
19. Krieger LM, Krieger AJ. The intercostal to phrenic nerve transfer: an effective means of reanimating the diaphragm in patients with high cervical spine injury. Plast Reconstr Surg 2000;105:1255–61.
20. DiMarco AF. Respiratory muscle stimulation in patients with spinal cord injury. In: Horch KW, Dhillon GS, editors. Neuroprosthetics: Theory and Practice. Hackensack, NJ: World Scientific; 2004. p. 951–78.
21. DiMarco AF, Takaoka Y, Kowalski KE. Combined intercostal and diaphragm pacing to provide artificial ventilation in patients with tetraplegia. Arch Phys Med Rehabil 2005;86:1200–7.

Functional Electrical Stimulation and Spinal Cord Injury

Chester H. Ho, MD[a],*, Ronald J. Triolo, PhD[b,c,d,e],
Anastasia L. Elias, PhD[f], Kevin L. Kilgore, PhD[d,e,g,h],
Anthony F. DiMarco, MD[e,h], Kath Bogie, DPhil[b,c,d,g],
Albert H. Vette, PhD[i,j], Musa L. Audu, PhD[b,d], Rudi Kobetic, MS[b],
Sarah R. Chang, BS[b,d], K. Ming Chan, MD[k],
Sean Dukelow, MD, PhD[a], Dennis J. Bourbeau, PhD[g,h],
Steven W. Brose, DO[g,h,l], Kenneth J. Gustafson, PhD[d,g,h],
Zelma H.T. Kiss, MD, PhD[m], Vivian K. Mushahwar, PhD[k]

KEYWORDS

- Electric stimulation • Electrodes • Spinal cord injuries • Rehabilitation
- Muscle spasticity • Pressure ulcer • Neurogenic urinary bladder • Paralysis

[a] Division of Physical Medicine & Rehabilitation, Department of Clinical Neurosciences, Foothills Medical Centre, Room 1195, 1403-29th Street NW, Calgary, Alberta T2N 2T9, Canada; [b] Louis Stokes Cleveland VA Medical Center, Advanced Platform Technology Center, 151 AW/APT, 10701 East Boulevard, Cleveland, OH 44106, USA; [c] Department of Orthopaedics, Case Western Reserve University, MetroHealth Medical Center, 2500 MetroHealth Drive, Cleveland, OH 44109, USA; [d] Department of Biomedical Engineering, Case Western Reserve University, 10900 Euclid Avenue, Cleveland, OH 44106, USA; [e] MetroHealth Medical Center, 2500 MetroHealth Drive, Cleveland, OH 44109, USA; [f] Chemical and Materials Engineering, W7-002 ECERF, University of Alberta, Edmonton, Alberta T6G 2V4, Canada; [g] Louis Stokes Cleveland VA Medical Center, 10701 East Boulevard, Cleveland, OH 44106, USA; [h] Cleveland FES Center, 11000 Cedar Avenue, Suite 230, Cleveland, OH 44106-3056, USA; [i] Department of Mechanical Engineering, University of Alberta, 4-9 Mechanical Engineering Building, Edmonton, Alberta T6G 2G8, Canada; [j] Glenrose Rehabilitation Hospital, Alberta Health Services, 10230 - 111 Avenue, Edmonton, Alberta T5G 0B7, Canada; [k] Division of Physical Medicine and Rehabilitation, Centre for Neuroscience, University of Alberta, 5005 Katz Group Centre, 11361-87 Avenue, Edmonton, Alberta T6G 2E1, Canada; [l] Ohio University Heritage College of Osteopathic Medicine, Grosvenor Hall, Athens, OH 45701, USA; [m] Department of Clinical Neurosciences, Foothills Medical Centre, Room 1195, 1403-29th Street NW, Calgary, Alberta T2N 2T9, Canada
* Corresponding author.
E-mail address: chester.ho@albertahealthservices.ca

Phys Med Rehabil Clin N Am 25 (2014) 631–654
http://dx.doi.org/10.1016/j.pmr.2014.05.001
1047-9651/14/$ – see front matter © 2014 Elsevier Inc. All rights reserved.

KEY POINTS

- Functional electrical stimulation (FES) of the peripheral and central nervous system may be used for rehabilitation and management of complications after spinal cord injury (SCI).
- FES may improve the functional status and quality of life of many persons with spinal cord injuries.
- Many of the FES strategies are already commercially available, whereas others are being tested in human and laboratory studies.
- FES should be routinely considered as part of the rehabilitation and medical management of eligible persons with spinal cord injuries.

An injury to the spinal cord can disrupt communications between the brain and body, leading to a loss of control over otherwise intact neuromuscular systems. By taking advantage of these intact neuromuscular systems, several neuroprostheses have been developed to restore functions through functional electrical stimulation (FES) of the central and peripheral nervous system. Neuroprostheses using FES to control the paralyzed muscles may prevent many secondary medical complications and improve functional independence by providing a means to exercise and negotiate physical barriers. Improvements in multiple body systems and functions have been reported through the use of FES, and they are discussed in this article. These devices range in complexity and include components such as power supplies (which may be completely external to the body or implanted and recharged with radio frequency waves), a control circuit (ie, the brains of the device), lead wires, connectors, external braces, and sensors. This article describes the basic properties of the electrodes, the current FES system being developed in research and in clinical practice, and the future of these devices.

THE BASIC PROPERTIES OF ELECTRODES FOR NERVE STIMULATION

In neuroprostheses, electrodes are the interface between the external circuitry and the tissue, delivering a charge that stimulates the nerves connected to the muscles of interest. This charge perturbs the resting potential of the neuron (typically around −65 mV); if this value is raised beyond a threshold, membrane depolarization occurs. This depolarization results in an influx of Na^+ ions, initiating an action potential that can travel spatially down the length of an axon. A coordinated group of action potentials can lead to a muscle contraction.[1] By targeting nerves rather than the muscle fibers themselves (which can also be stimulated electrically), substantially smaller charge densities may be used, consuming less power and avoiding tissue damage.[2]

Provided that the neuromuscular system is intact, stimulation may be achieved at a variety of locations (from the origin of the neuron in the spinal cord to the peripheral nerve and to the skin above the muscle) using various types of electrodes. The simplest configuration uses large (of the order of square centimeters) electrodes placed on the surface of the skin. The electrodes are easily replaced; however, achieving accurate and precise positioning is challenging, and charge is distributed over a large area. A more invasive approach is to implant needlelike electrodes percutaneously into the muscle of interest. This method is considered a precursor to fully implanted systems, although subcutaneous electrodes themselves can remain functional for years.[3] When electrodes are fully implanted in close proximity to the nerve, even more precise targeting can be achieved using even smaller current densities, which are less likely to damage the tissue.

Electrodes have been designed to wrap around individual nerves, with a range of geometries, including spiral,[4] helical,[5] and rectangular.[6] To selectively address smaller groups of axons within a nerve and to reach areas that are not readily accessible from the surface, intrafascicular electrodes may be inserted into the nerve itself.[7] Pools of neurons may also be stimulated directly in the spinal cord in intraspinal microstimulation (ISMS).[8] Although implanted devices offer superior targeting, the obvious drawback is the invasiveness of the insertion process and the potential risk of infection, although this has not been reported as a significant issue.[9]

In FES, the electrode typically acts as a conductor, delivering electrical charge from a power supply to the tissue. Charge transfer occurs when voltage applied between the active electrode and a second electrode (called the reference electrode) generates an electric field, which in turn forces electrical charge to flow. In systems in which multiple stimulation channels are used, a single reference electrode may be used. When a voltage is applied, the energy can drive several unwanted chemical reactions. To avoid generating H_2 gas from water, the voltage generated between the electrodes must not exceed the amount required to electrolyze water (-0.6 V to -0.8 V depending on electrode type[10]). The amount of charge that can be delivered within these limits depends on the impedance of the material, which should be low to maximize the current delivered. To balance the charge injected to stimulate the neurons and prevent the electrochemical decomposition of tissue, a secondary pulse of opposite polarity should be included in the stimulation profile (ie, a biphasic pulse should be applied). The electrodes themselves must be selected to be resistant to corrosion under physiologic conditions, even under an applied voltage. Common electrode materials for implanted devices include corrosion-resistant stainless steel and noble metals such as PtIr or Pt (which have highly stable atomic configurations and therefore are resistant to chemical processes such as corrosion or oxidation). Other metals (including silver, iron, and copper) are known to elicit dramatic inflammatory response in vivo and should be avoided.[11]

The time-dependent failure of neural interfaces in vivo is an impediment to long-term use, particularly for recording electrodes and stimulating electrodes, which inject small currents into small target areas. The principal cause of failure of these devices is the encapsulation, which occurs as a part of the foreign body response, insulating the electrodes from their surroundings.[12] To avoid scar formation initiated by mechanical mismatch between stiff electrodes and soft tissues, there is an increasing interest in fabricating electrodes and arrays from soft (low modulus) materials such as silicone elastomer.[13] Beyond this, several strategies have been undertaken to modify the surface properties of electrodes to improve the interactions that take place with surrounding tissue and reduce glial scar formation.[14] When developing new electrodes, arrays, and coatings, in vitro testing may be used initially to screen the cellular response, but they must be tested in vivo following the standard ISO 10993.

UPPER EXTREMITY FUNCTIONAL RESTORATION WITH FES

For persons with cervical-level SCI, restoration of hand function is their top priority.[15] Neuroprostheses using FES provide the most promising method for significant gain in hand and arm function for this population. Muscle contractions can be orchestrated to produce coordinated grasp opening and closing; thumb opening, closing, and positioning; wrist extension and flexion; forearm pronation; and elbow extension for persons with C5-C6–level SCI. Neuroprostheses can be coupled with tendon transfers to maximize function.[16] The objectives of these neuroprostheses are to reduce the need to rely on assistance from others; the need for adaptive equipment, braces, or other orthotic devices; and the time it takes to perform tasks. Neuroprostheses make use of the patient's own paralyzed musculature to provide the power for grasp and the patient's voluntary musculature to control the grasp. Typically, persons with SCI use the neuroprosthesis for eating, personal hygiene, writing, and office tasks.

Neuroprostheses have been clinically implemented and investigated using systems based on surface electrodes, percutaneous electrodes, and implanted devices. Surface and percutaneous systems have potential application in muscle conditioning and in short-term research or clinical applications.[17] Implanted systems are generally used for long-term functional enhancement.

All existing upper extremity neuroprosthetic systems consist of (1) a stimulator that activates the muscles of the forearm and hand and (2) an input transducer and control unit. The control signal for grasp is derived from an action that the user has retained voluntary control over, which can include joint movement, muscle activity, respiration, or voice control.[18] A coordinated stimulation pattern is developed so that the muscles are activated in a sequence that produces a functional grasp pattern as the user typically has control over grasp opening and closing but does not have direct control over the activation of each muscle.

Surface stimulation of the forearm and hand can be used to exercise and to produce functional movements. Nathan[19] developed a splint that incorporates surface electrodes for grasp. This system is commercially available (NESS H200, Bioness, Valencia, CA, USA) and is primarily intended for therapeutic applications after stroke or SCI, such as building muscle strength, preventing joint contractures, and improving tissue viability. Popovic and colleagues[20] have developed a surface stimulation system called the ETHZ-ParaCare neuroprosthesis. This system is capable of 4 channels of stimulation and can be interfaced with a variety of control inputs. Early functional results indicate that subjects can use the system to perform a variety of activities of daily living (ADL) in the home.[21]

Implanted FES systems have been used for long-term functional enhancement for persons with cervical SCI. The largest clinical trial of an upper extremity neuroprosthesis was the Freehand trial, initiated by the Cleveland Functional Electrical Stimulation Center in 1992.[22] The Freehand neuroprosthesis used an implanted 8-channel receiver-stimulator, and control of grasp opening and closing was achieved through graded elevation of the user's contralateral shoulder. Using the neuroprosthesis, 100% of the participants ($n = 28$) improved in independence in at least 1 task, and 78% were less dependent in at least 3 tasks. More than 90% were satisfied with the neuroprosthesis.[23] The Freehand system was transferred to industry (NeuroControl Corp, Elyria, OH, USA) and was implemented successfully in more than 200 patients with SCI using neuroprostheses.[24] Despite the clinical success, the company exited the SCI market in 2001 and no longer markets the Freehand System.

A second-generation implanted neuroprosthesis has been developed, improving on the features of the Freehand System.[25] This system, called the Implanted Stimulator Telemeter Twelve-channel System (IST-12), has 12 stimulation channels and 2 channels of myoelectric signal recording acquisition.[26] To date, 12 subjects with SCI have been implanted with the IST-12 system, including 3 subjects with systems for restoring movement in both hands. Subjects successfully use the processed myoelectric signal from a wrist extensor for proportional control of grasp opening and closing. Every subject has demonstrated improvement in at least 2 activities and as many as 11 activities. Most commonly, improvement was demonstrated in eating with a fork and writing with a pen. Other tasks in which subjects showed improvement included office tasks, using a cell phone, getting money out of a wallet, and embroidery,[25] as illustrated in **Fig. 1**.

Availability

At present, commercially available FES systems for grasp function in cervical SCI are limited to surface stimulation systems. Specifically, the NESS H200 is available by pre-scription at multiple sites throughout the world (www.bioness.com). Other systems, such as the Compex system, are primarily targeted for exercise training rather than function benefit. Efforts are underway to increase the availability of implanted neuro-prostheses to persons with SCI (http://casemed.case.edu/ifr/).

Future Directions

Future directions for FES hand systems include the development of fully implanted systems that eliminate the need to don and doff components[27] and the expanded use of myoelectric control algorithms to control multiple functions at the same time.[28] The use of signals derived directly from the brain (brain-computer interface), either externally or through implanted electrodes, is expected to result in more natural hand system control.[29] In addition, systems are being developed to provide whole-arm function for those with C4 or higher SCI.[30]

LOWER EXTREMITY FUNCTIONAL RESTORATION WITH FES

In persons with SCI, the inability to stand or step significantly limits the performance of many ADL such as washing dishes at a counter or reaching items on high shelves. For persons with thoracic-level complete SCI, stimulated contractions of the lower extremity muscles can enable standing and stepping, increase personal mobility, and improve general health and quality of life.[31] In persons with incomplete injuries, walking performance can be improved.[32]

Eight channels of continuous stimulation to the knee, hip, and trunk extensors can power the sit-to-stand transition and support the body vertically against collapse (**Fig. 2**).[33] Stimulation to the hip ab/adductors and ankle plantar/dorsiflexors has been included in experimental systems for sensor-based control of standing balance in the coronal and sagittal planes.[34] Existing neuroprostheses for lower extremity func-tion use maximal levels of constant stimulation at the hips and knees.[35] Recipients of a neuroprosthesis with epimysial and intramuscular electrodes that continuously acti-vated the vasti, gluteals, hamstrings, and lumbar erector spinae exhibited mean and median standing times of 10 and 3 minutes, respectively.[33] This time is sufficient for facilitating transfers to high surfaces, performing swing-to gait for short distances in wheelchair-inaccessible environments, and participating in other social, work, and personal activities. Some implant recipients in a phase II clinical trial of the system were able to stand for more than 20 minutes, and all were able to release 1 hand from a walker or assistive device to reach objects overhead (**Fig. 3**). On average, 90% of body weight was placed on the legs, reducing requirements on the arms to only light touch to maintain balance. System performance and patterns of usage were maintained after discharge for at least 1 year of follow-up. Although there were no discernible interactions between injury level, degree of preserved sensation, or time postinjury and system performance, outcomes seem to be inversely propor-tional to height and weight, implying that body mass index may be an important clinical factor for determining expectations.[35] Long-term use of neuroprostheses for standing was safe and effective and had no adverse physiologic effects.

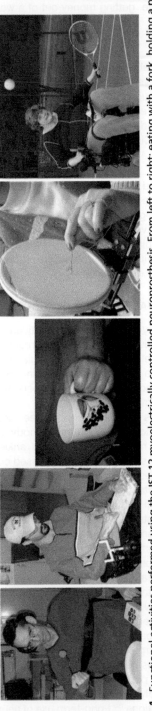

Fig. 1. Functional activities performed using the IST-12 myoelectrically controlled neuroprosthesis. From left to right: eating with a fork, holding a pen to write, holding a cup, needle embroidery, holding a tennis racquet.

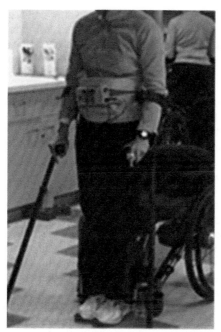

Fig. 2. Implant recipient (C7 AIS C) standing with FES to the knee, hip, and trunk extensors, and hip/trunk ab/adductors. Multicontact cuff electrodes on the femoral nerves selectively activate the uniarticular heads of the quadriceps (vastus lateralis, intermedius, and medialis).

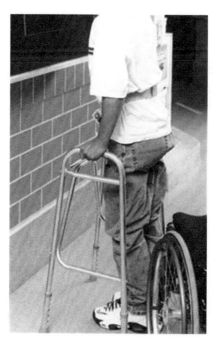

Fig. 3. Eight-channel implant recipient (T9 AIS A) releases one hand for overhead reaching activities while standing with the neuroprosthesis.

Stepping of up to 100 m has also been achieved after paralysis with simple preprogrammed patterns of open-loop stimulation delivered from the surface or via 8- and 16-channel implanted pulse generators.[36] Once initiated by the user, stepping motions can cycle continuously while the appropriate adjustments are made with the upper body until the pattern is stopped. Alternatively, the stimulation for sequential steps can be triggered from successive depressions of ring- or walker-mounted switches or automatically from body-mounted sensors, such as inclinometers, accelerometers, gyroscopes, or foot or heel switches.[37] The largest potential impact of stimulation may be for people with motor incomplete injuries (**Fig. 4**) who require activation of a small number of muscles during the gait cycle to become household or community ambulators.[38] In such cases, gait training with stimulation can have a therapeutic effect in terms of improved voluntary strength, walking speed, stride length, and cadence even after completion of aggressive conventional therapies.[39] Interactive use of stimulation to assist gait resulted consistently in an additional 20% improvement in walking speed and 6-minute distance, as well as a more than 3-fold increase in maximum walking distance, illustrating a significant neuroprosthetic effect. Walking with stimulation was also more dynamic as evidenced by decreased time spent in the double support phases of gait. The electromyographic activity of muscles under volitional control has also been exploited as a command source to control stimulation in persons with incomplete injuries, which has the potential to coordinate stimulated contractions with voluntary motor function, and in so doing reinforce voluntary movement patterns and provide a mechanism to continuously modulate walking speed and cadence.[40]

Surface FES to the lower extremity muscles with intact innervation has allowed cycling movement that simulates exercise training, leading to increase in oxygen consumption during exercise,[41] muscle mass and strength, and quality of life in persons with chronic SCI.[42]

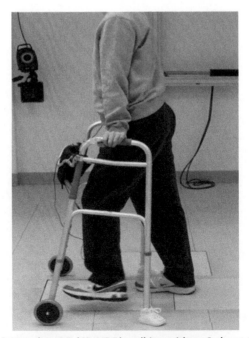

Fig. 4. Subject with incomplete SCI (C5 AIS D) walking with an 8-channel implanted receiver stimulator for activation of hip flexors and ankle dorsiflexors.

Availability

Although implanted standing and walking systems clearly provide significant functional and clinical benefits, such systems are only available on a research basis. Limited lower extremity function is possible with commercially available surface stimulators with reduced channel counts.[43]

FES cycling devices are available through Restorative Therapies, Inc. (www.restorative-therapies.com) and Therapeutic Alliances, Inc. (www.musclepower.com) in the United States.

Future Directions

Standing performance with implanted neuroprostheses can be improved significantly by using nerve-based electrodes, which more fully recruit the target muscles. Continuous stimulation of the femoral nerve with a multicontact cuff electrode below the branches to the rectus femoris and sartorius was shown to extend standing time and accelerate progress through reconditioning rehabilitation and balance training with the system.[44] The potential to delay the effects of fatigue by alternating activation of independent motor unit pools within a muscle via multicontact nerve cuffs or multiple independent nerve- or muscle-based electrodes is also being investigated.[45] At present, neuroprostheses are generally unresponsive to environmental disturbances, necessitating use of the arms for balance on an assistive device. Additional research is also focusing on automatically modulating stimulation in response to perturbations to reduce reliance on the upper extremities, allow users to alter their postures in advance of anticipated disturbances, and minimize the risk of falls while standing or using advanced biomechanical modeling techniques to optimize stimulus patterns during walking or while assuming various task-dependent standing postures.[46] Another promising development involves the combination of FES with exoskeletal bracing that can lock, unlock, or couple the joints as necessary to avoid fatigue and smoothly shape limb trajectories or that can inject small amounts of assistive power when the stimulated responses are too weak or fatigued to complete a motion.[47] With such an approach, users would be able to walk under their own power and therefore accrue the physiologic benefits of exercising the paralyzed muscles in addition to those of standing, weight bearing, and mobilization.

TRUNK CONTROL AND POSTURE WITH FES

After SCI, trunk muscles can oftentimes not provide the necessary forces to adequately control trunk posture because of a lack of innervation[48] and/or muscle atrophy,[49] significantly limiting their performance during ADL[50] and even leading to secondary health complications such as reduced respiratory capacity.[51] To compensate for insufficient muscle control during sitting, persons with SCI usually tilt their pelvis further backward to increase stability in the anterior direction.[52] When reaching, they oftentimes use one arm thrown over the back of their chair to provide the external forces necessary to keep the trunk from bending forward uncontrollably. Compensational sitting arrangements can, however, lead to kyphosis[52] and pressure ulcers (PUs) that arise from asymmetric trunk orientation and infrequent weight redistribution. It is therefore not surprising that persons with SCI have prioritized the recovery of trunk control over the recovery of walking function and other essential functional abilities.[15]

Bracing devices such as corsets are perhaps the most common items for stabilizing the trunk after SCI. To improve reaching and wheelchair propulsion, some persons with SCI use chest straps.[53] In the general case of reaching from a wheelchair during ADL, chest straps or other restraints are highly undesirable as they hinder free and spontaneous movement, decrease available trunk range of motion, and draw undue attention to themselves. Other studies have shown that the large forces exerted on the abdomen by a fabric corset might cause abnormal increases in the intra-abdominal pressure, potentially leading to disturbance of the viscera.[54]

Stiffening the paralyzed trunk and hip extensors with continuous FES has a multitude of benefits: it can correct kyphotic seated postures, normalize lateral vertebral alignment, improve ventilation and respiratory volumes, and alter interface pressures.[55] It can also expand bimanual workspace,[48] statically stabilize the torso (**Fig. 5**), increase the forces that can be exerted on objects with the upper extremities, return users to erect sitting from a fully forward-flexed posture, and improve manual wheelchair propulsion efficiency at comfortable speeds.[56] Independent bed turning and wheelchair transfers can also be facilitated by more rigidly coupling the pelvis to the shoulders when the paralyzed core trunk muscles are continuously activated with stimulation to stiffen the torso.[57] In addition, activating the quadratus lumborum with surface or implanted electrodes has been shown to enhance mediolateral stability and assist with attaining side leaning postures, whereas coactivation with the abdominal muscles can further stiffen the trunk while seated or assist in attaining forward leaning postures. Some of the required muscles to achieve these clinical outcomes can be accessed via surface stimulation; however, strong and isolated contractions are robustly and repeatably achieved by exciting the T12-L2 spinal nerves associated with the lumbar erector spinae and other muscles (**Fig. 6**) using intramuscular electrodes and surgically implanted pulse generators.[58] The strategy of continuously activating the core trunk and hip muscles only substitutes one statically stable posture for another. Upper extremity effort is still required to stabilize the body during transitions between nonstimulated and stimulated postures and to maintain balance or restore erect sitting when exposed to internal or external perturbations.

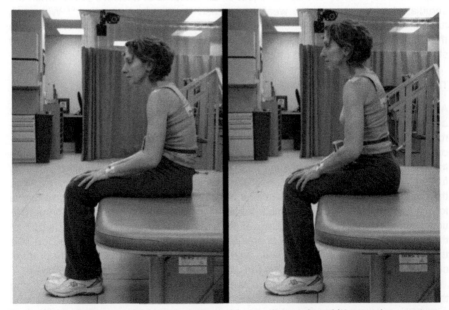

Fig. 5. Effect of FES on seated posture. By stimulating the trunk and hip muscles, consistent significant changes in posterior pelvic tilt and shoulder height were recorded.

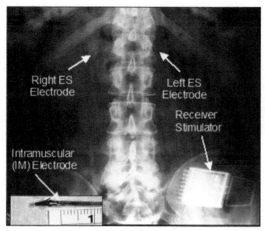

Fig. 6. Radiograph of an implanted trunk system showing intramuscular electrodes (*inset*) inserted into T12-L1 to activate the lumbar erector spinae muscles.

Extensive studies have been carried out to assess the strategy used by the intact central nervous system to mediate trunk balance in neurologically intact persons. Such studies mainly involve biomechanical simulations and experimental observations of the static and dynamic behaviors of trunk posture in a seated pose.[59] These studies confirmed the initial feasibility of using continuous stimulation to increase trunk stiffness, vary trunk posture, and resist static perturbations. Moreover, they resulted in tools for evaluating more sophisticated control systems that might allow users to set their own task-dependent postures and maintain balance during internal or external perturbations. Studies have established the feasibility of a self-righting control system that works on the dynamic movement of the trunk to automatically return to an erect posture from forward-flexed positions by monitoring trunk tilt and modulating stimulation to the trunk and hip extensors appropriately (**Fig. 7**).[60] In this study, 5 persons with SCI volunteered to test a simple threshold-based set-point controller. The controller worked consistently across all subjects despite considerable intersubject variability in terms of SCI level and motor and sensory impairment.

Availability

At present, neuroprostheses for controlling the paralyzed torso and enhancing seated function can be obtained only through research and development studies, whereas attempts to commercialize such systems are ongoing.

Future Directions

Advanced systems to control seated posture and trunk balance have the potential to prevent falls from the wheelchair while performing ADL, during sudden collisions and unexpected stops, and while negotiating bumpy or uneven terrain, thus eliminating the need for chest straps or other constraints that would hinder function. New systems that can sense trunk and wheelchair positions, velocity, or acceleration, as well as communicate the user's intent to closed-loop controllers need to be developed. Important requirements of such systems are that they are portable, appear natural, and can be easily integrated with any residual motor and/or sensory function. Such systems also need to be translated into routine clinical use and disseminated widely

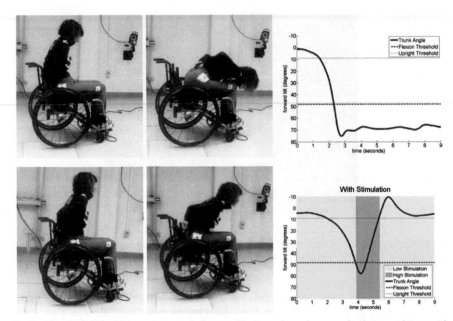

Fig. 7. Simple threshold-based control of seated balance based on trunk tilt in a subject with C8 tetraplegia. Without stimulation (*top*) of the hip and trunk extensors, the subject cannot return to erect sitting from a fully forward-flexed position without use of the arms. With the controller active (*bottom*), forward trunk tilt is arrested before a forward fall, and upright posture is automatically restored.

in home and community environments. Future directions also include the timing of the stimulation to coincide with different phases of the manual wheelchair propulsion cycle to improve efficiency during ramp ascent or varying speeds, utilization during rowing exercise, and early introduction of trunk control systems soon after injury to prevent the development of spinal deformities and help vary posture to augment pressure relief maneuvers.

FES TECHNIQUES TO RESTORE RESPIRATORY MUSCLE FUNCTION

The use of FES to improve respiratory muscle function is discussed in depth in the article by Dalal and DiMarco elsewhere in this issue.

PREVENTION OF PRESSURE ULCERS THROUGH FUNCTIONAL ELECTRICAL STIMULATION

PUs are a common complication after SCI. They cause psychological distress, have a detrimental effect on quality of life, and place a significant burden on health care systems, with costs estimated at $6 to $15 billion per year in the United States.[61] Preventing PUs from developing in the first place reduces patient suffering, improves patient outcomes and quality of life, and reduces the large health care costs associated with treating them. Indeed, it has been estimated that prevention of PUs is approximately 2.5 times more economical than treating them.[62]

PUs can develop in one of 2 ways. They can originate at the surface of the skin and progress inward if unattended. Skin inspections are often effective in detecting these ulcers at an early stage of development. If unattended, these ulcers can progressively affect deeper tissue layers ending at the bone. PUs can also originate at deep muscle-bone interfaces and progress outward. These ulcers have only recently been acknowledged clinically and are now referred to as deep tissue injury (DTI). Sustained pressure leads to unrelieved mechanical deformation, tissue ischemia, and ischemia-reperfusion injury. Muscle is more susceptible to breakdown because of mechanical deformation and ischemia-reperfusion injury than skin; thus, damage originates within muscle tissue around bony prominences much sooner than in the skin. Skin inspections are ineffective in detecting DTI at their earliest stages of development, and there are no clinically viable methods for the early detection of DTI. Therefore, these ulcers often develop unbeknownst to the affected individual or their caregiver. Once DTIs exhibit obvious skin signs, for example, purple discoloration, extensive damage in the underlying soft tissue had already occurred. Prevention strategies such as pressure redistributing surfaces (mattresses and seating cushions) and periodical weight shifts have not decreased the incidence of PU; in fact, with the improved awareness of DTI, the prevalence of PU is on the rise.[63] Other approaches to prevent PU are necessary. FES through surface stimulation and implanted electrodes are two novel ways to prevent PU, each having their own specific advantages and disadvantages. Both systems require intact innervation to the gluteal muscles.

Intermittent Electrical Stimulation for the Prevention of DTI

Intermittent electrical stimulation[64] (IES) was developed for the prevention of DTI. This method applies brief electrical stimulation through surface electrodes to muscles around bony prominences that are loaded during sitting or lying down (eg, the gluteus maximus muscles) every few minutes causing them to contract. These periodical contractions mimic the subconscious postural adjustments conducted by able-bodied persons in response to discomfort while sitting or lying down. Ten seconds of IES causing fused muscle contractions in the gluteus muscles every 10 minutes while sitting redistribute surface pressure away from the ischial tuberosities and increase tissue oxygenation in study participants independently of gluteal muscle mass.[65,66] Moreover, IES-induced contractions significantly redistribute internal pressure away from the bony prominences[67] and reduce tissue deformation in the muscles between the ischial tuberosity and skin even when loading levels as high as 75% of body weight in adult pigs with SCI were applied.[67] IES is effective in significantly reducing or completely eliminating the formation of DTI in adult rats and pigs,[68] thus establishing a strong scientific support for the utility of IES as a means for preventing DTI in clinical settings.

Implanted Neuromuscular Stimulation for Tissue Health and Pressure Ulcer Prevention

Another approach of FES for PU prevention is through stimulation of the inferior gluteal nerve, which innervates the gluteus maximus muscle and lies deep to the buttock surface and close to the sciatic nerve. Surface electrode placement for preferential recruitment of the inferior gluteal nerve can be difficult for users to achieve. Moreover, repeatable electrode placement in the upper buttock region may be hard to accomplish for either independent users or their carers. Implanted neuromuscular electrical stimulation (NMES) systems for long-term therapeutic use have dual advantages. The stimulating tip of the electrode can be located close to the motor point of the nerve of interest; this reduces the charge required to elicit a contractile response and ensures that the response is repeatable and predicable. The user does not have to replace the stimulating electrode every day, so the system is both reliable and simple to use.

The gluteal stimulation v1 (GSTIM I) system using implanted electrodes with percutaneous leads provides both concurrent bilateral and alternating gluteal stimulation to deliver muscle conditioning and regular weight shifting to the user. GSTIM I has been shown to have a positive impact on multiple aspects of tissue health. Subjects who received GSTIM I have shown statistically significant changes between baseline and postintervention ischial region interface pressure (**Fig. 8**). Maximum gluteal muscle thickness significantly increased and was maintained with regular use of gluteal NMES.[69] Tissue oxygen levels also improved with regular use of dynamic stimulation but decreased on withdrawal.

In addition to the long-term changes in muscle characteristics, weight shifting induced by gluteal NMES dynamically alters conditions at the seating support interface facilitated by stimulated muscular contractions. This dynamic effect increases over time as the paralyzed muscles become stronger with regular use of implanted gluteal NMES. Chronic application of gluteal stimulation is thus uniquely able to affect the intrinsic properties of paralyzed muscle through contractile responses to repeated stimulation, increasing muscle thickness and blood flow together with reducing regional interface pressures.[70,71] Use of GSTIM I also increased sitting tolerance and minimized the impact of minor incidents such as skin tears due to poor transfers, which were reported to be resolved in days rather than in weeks.

Therapeutic implanted NMES provides a unique intrinsic approach to reducing the risk of PU development for persons with SCI. Daily use of NMES is indicated to

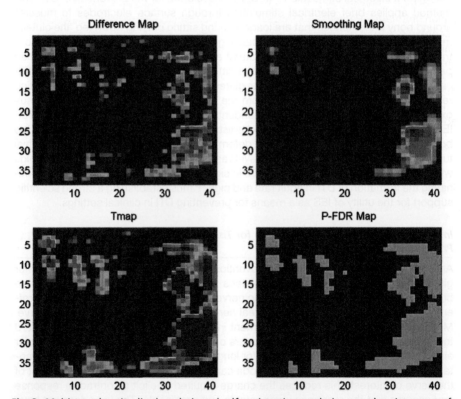

Fig. 8. Multistage longitudinal analysis and self-registration analysis maps showing areas of significant change in seated interface pressures over time (output adjusted for simultaneous testing at multiple locations).

maintain hypertrophy of paralyzed muscles. Long-term use of gluteal NMES using implanted systems may provide an adjunctive method to ensure a regular pressure-relief regimen in high-risk persons, which can reduce the risk of PU development and allow users to participate more fully in ADL.

Availability

Both the IES system and the fully implanted NMES for the prevention of PUs are under research protocol use only.

Future Directions

Further research is underway to examine the efficacy and effectiveness of the approach for PU prevention with both the surface stimulation and implanted systems. A system for clinical use to deliver IES to the gluteal region, known as Smart-e-Pants[72] (Smart-electronic-Pants) **(Fig. 9)**, was developed. It is composed of a garment, surface electrodes, and a small battery-operated stimulator. The electrodes are placed on mesh panels in the garment. Safety, feasibility, and acceptability of Smart-e-Pants have been tested in a wide range of health care settings, including 50 volunteers in an acute rehabilitation unit, tertiary rehabilitation hospital, a long-term care facility, and home care. Study participants used the system for at least 4 weeks, 12 hours per day. The system proved to be safe and feasible in all 4 clinical settings. No PU was observed in any of the participants. Donning and doffing of the Smart-e-Pants system took between 7 and 18 minutes. Patients and caregivers did not find the application of Smart-e-Pants or IES to be disruptive and indicated that the stimulation was acceptable as part of their daily routine in more than 97% of the time. These preliminary clinical studies on IES as a preventative treatment strategy are promising. Studies are currently underway to test the effectiveness of the IES approach in preventing pressure ulcers, and demonstrate the improvements in health and cost outcomes that it may provide.

Future development of the fully implanted NMES system will use a small, rechargeable stimulator customized to provide 2 synchronized channels of stimulation to

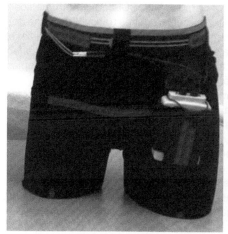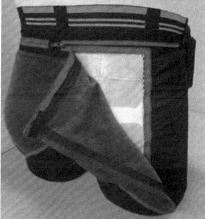

Fig. 9. Smart-e-pants system showing garment, mesh panel for surface electrodes, and stimulator. (*Courtesy of* Project Sensory Motor Adaptive Rehabilitation Technology (SMART), Edmonton, Alberta, Canada; with permission.)

automatically produce the regular weight-shift maneuvers recommended for periodic pressure relief when seated in the wheelchair.

FES FOR RESTORING BLADDER CONTROL

The lower urinary tract (LUT) functions in the storage and emptying of urine. After SCI with an upper motor neuron injury to the sacral nerve roots, volitional control of these functions is frequently lost and the LUT becomes hyperreflexive. Incontinence can occur when the detrusor produces large, uninhibited reflex contractions at low volumes of stored urine. Simultaneously with detrusor contractions, the external urethral sphincter (EUS) may reflexively contract as pressure builds in the urethra during voiding, producing detrusor-sphincter dyssynergia (DSD). This uncoordinated reflex and the subsequent high bladder pressures can result in inefficient voiding, incontinence, and ureteric reflux, causing renal injury. In addition, DSD can also cause autonomic dysreflexia (AD), which can be life-threatening if not resolved. Finally, loss of bladder control has a severe impact on quality of life and self-image. Persons with SCI list bladder function restoration among the highest priority for restoration, more than standing and ambulation.[15]

Persons with SCI frequently report ineffectiveness with existing bladder management, medication side effects, challenges associated with bladder catheterization strategies, and complications associated with surgical solutions. Similar to many other complications of SCI discussed earlier, there remains a critically unmet need to restore bladder function lost to SCI and the use of FES may offer an effective solution.

FES offers a means to restore LUT function by activating the bladder and inhibiting the urethral sphincter to produce voiding or by inhibiting the bladder to provide urinary continence and reduce triggers for AD and restore LUT function.[73] The Brindley approach was the first widely clinically available FES system for bladder function.[74] This approach produces bladder contractions by stimulating bladder motor efferents in the sacral roots. To avoid cocontraction of the EUS and detrusor preventing fluid flow, stimulation is delivered in repeated bursts. After each burst, the striated EUS muscle relaxes, but the smooth-muscle bladder relaxes more slowly, maintaining bladder pressure and creating a pressure gradient that causes poststimulus urine flow. This system has been implanted in thousands of persons with SCI and is both medically effective and cost-effective.[75] However, this approach requires transection of the dorsal spinal roots (dorsal rhizotomy) to eliminate unwanted bladder and urethral reflexes due to sensory feedback. This rhizotomy also eliminates desirable reflexes that affect sexual and bowel functions and removes the opportunity for future clinical therapies, markedly reducing acceptance of this approach by persons with SCI.[76]

Stimulation of peripheral sensory pathways can access and influence the spinal neural circuits that control pelvic reflexes and function. Afferent-mediated neural prostheses take advantage of natural nervous system processes and are potentially less invasive than spinal-root-based approaches such as the Brindley system. This approach has the potential to provide more natural function than motor-driven approaches, although it is more dependent on stimulation patterns and other inputs to the spinal circuits. One such approach uses genital nerve stimulation to achieve direct spinal level bladder inhibition. This approach has primarily been applied for immediate use, but it has also shown to improve urinary continence and bladder capacity in persons with SCI during short-duration use.[77,78] If longer-term use is effective, then this approach may provide both a noninvasive and implanted option. Bladder inhibition via implanted electrodes on the pudendal nerve[79] and sacral roots[80] can also provide bladder inhibition in persons with SCI.

Availability

There are several neural prostheses in development to restore pelvic functions for persons with SCI to activate or inhibit the bladder and urethral sphincter and provide a rhizotomy-free Brindley system. They are not commercially available yet.

Future Directions

Some approaches have been shown to be effective in animal models and may be promising for human studies. Bladder activation and voiding via pudendal urethral afferent stimulation has been demonstrated in animal models, and human studies suggest that bladder excitation can be achieved.[81] This approach may provide a peripheral-based alternative to sacral-root-based bladder activation.

Urethral sphincter inhibition and bladder voiding can be obtained with patterned afferent stimulation of sacral dermatomes.[82] This approach has achieved clinical daily voiding of awake animals with chronic SCI. It may potentially provide a less-invasive alternative in humans. Finally, high-frequency (kilohertz) stimulation can provide temporary, reversible, and complete conduction block of the pudendal nerve, and thus stop reflexive EUS contractions, allowing bladder voiding equivalent to nerve transection.[83] Bilateral pudendal nerve block can provide clinical daily voiding of awake animals with chronic SCI. If this approach is effective in humans, it could be combined with pudendal bladder inhibition to restore bladder function with a single implant.

INTRASPINAL MICROSTIMULATION FOR GAIT RESTORATION

Apart from the aforementioned systems that are either commercially available or closer to clinical availability, one novel experimental approach is worth noting. A significant limitation of the surface stimulation system to restore walking is that many of the key muscles required for walking lie deep in the leg and are not accessible with surface electrodes. Even with the percutaneous implantation system, many channels are required to stimulate these different muscles. Mushahwar and colleagues [84–87] have pioneered the use of implanted electrodes in the spinal cord to overcome these problems. This approach, known as intraspinal microstimulation (ISMS), has shown promising results in pre-clinical animal studies. Intraspinal microstimulation entails the implantation of a few fine, hair-like wires in the ventral horns of the small lumbosacral enlargement of the spinal cord (~ 5 cm long in humans). This region contains the cell bodies of the motoneurons innervating all the muscles of the lower extremity, as well as large proportions of the neural networks involved in locomotion. Tapping into this region allows access to the standing and stepping control centre in the spinal cord. Stimulation through a single ISMS microwire can produce selective movements around one joint.[85,86,89] A single ISMS microwire can also activate synergistic muscle groups that produce coordinated multi-joint movements such as downward full limb extension, upward flexion, forward reaching, and backward propulsion,[87] which eliminates the need for routing electrodes widely through the body to each member of a muscle group producing these movements. The levels of stimulation with ISMS (<0.1 mA) are orders of magnitude less than those required for stimulation through the skin or percutaneous electrodes. Moreover, the levels required for generating functional limb movements generate no signs of discomfort or pain in conscious experimental animals implanted with ISMS microwires. By activating the underlying locomotor-related networks in the lumbosacral enlargement, ISMS activates the motoneurons trans-synaptically. This in turn recruits the motor units in a near normal physiological order which produces graded recruitment of force and large improvements in fatigue-resistance relative to FES systems targeting the muscles or peripheral nerves.[84,90] In chronically implanted animals, ISMS microwires remained stable throughout the duration of implantation and produced negligible damage in the spinal cord.[88,91] In adult cats, ISMS was effective in producing long durations of standing that, on average, were 5 times longer than durations produced by peripheral FES.[92] Moreover, ISMS produced long durations of in-place stepping in animals with chronic SCI and atrophied muscles.[93] In deeply anesthetized animals, ISMS was capable of producing long distances (>1 km) of weight-bearing and propulsive over-ground walking[94]; these distances were 10 times longer than walking distances produced by peripheral FES.[95] The produced walking was adaptable on-the fly using intelligent control strategies that adjusted the stimulation pattern based on miniature force and position sensors mounted on the legs.[95,96] The intelligent control strategies allowed for automatic adaptations to perturbations as well as muscle fatigue. Interestingly, both standing and walking with ISMS were produced with as few as 4 microwires in each side of the spinal cord.

Given the promising results obtained by ISMS, a proof-of-principle human study is currently planned, and a number of considerations are under discussion. These include patient selection, instrumentation, level of spinal cord injury, and fusion of spinal vertebra around the implant region. The most common sites of traumatic SCI are the cervical and thoracolumbar junction, while mid-thoracic injuries constitute 35% of all injuries. The appropriate volunteers for the study would be drawn from the mid-thoracic pool. While younger patients are generally better candidates for any experimental therapy, a temporary implant or an intra-operative mapping procedure to determine the ability of ISMS to produce functional leg movements may preclude these persons from undergoing permanent implantation in the future. Multiple penetrations of the spinal cord may result in gliosis, and opening the dura mater may produce a scar in the pia mater and arachnoid layers, making surgical re-exploration more difficult. Other surgical considerations include the ease of implanting very fine wires <100 μm in diameter into the spinal cord. Specialized instrumentation has been designed to inject stem cells successfully into the anterior horn of lumbar spinal segments[97,98] and could be adapted to insert electrodes as well. As with stem cell injection, anticipated complications include cerebrospinal fluid leakage. Minimally invasive insertion methods may be considered and fusion may be undertaken as part of the procedure to secure wires ema.

SUMMARY

Functional electrical stimulation has been well-studied and can be used in many ways to improve the well-being and functionality of persons with SCI. The scope of applications for FES in SCI continues to grow. Many options are commercially available both for institutional and home use, while others are still in research phase. When appropriate, SCI clinicians are encouraged to consider the use of FES as part of their standard regimen for rehabilitation or medical management of persons with SCI.

ACKNOWLEDGMENTS

The authors would like to thank the following institutions for their financial support: Alberta Innovates - Health Solutions, Canada Foundation for Innovation, Canadian Institutes of Health Research, Congressionally Directed and Peer-Reviewed Medical, Research Programs of the US Department of Defense (CDMRP/PRMRP), International Spinal Research Trust, National Institutes of Health (NIBIB and NINDS), Natural Sciences and Engineering Research Council of Canada, Project SMART, Rick Hansen

Man in Motion Fund, Spinal Cord Injury Treatment Centre Society, US Department of Defense Spinal Cord Injury Research Program, and US Department of Veterans Affairs Rehabilitation Research & Development Service.

REFERENCES

1. Popovic MR, Keller T, Papas IP, et al. Surface-stimulation technology for grasping and walking neuroprostheses. IEEE Eng Med Biol Mag 2001;20(1):82–93.
2. Ragnarsson KT. Functional electrical stimulation after spinal cord injury: current use, therapeutic effects and future directions. Spinal Cord 2007;46(4):255–74.
3. Agarwal S, Kobetic R, Nandurkar S, et al. Functional electrical stimulation for walking in paraplegia: 17-year follow-up of 2 cases. J Spinal Cord Med 2003; 26(1):86–91.
4. Naples GG, Mortimer JT, Scheiner A, et al. A spiral nerve cuff electrode for peripheral nerve stimulation. IEEE Trans Biomed Eng 1988;35:905–16.
5. Agnew WF, McCreery DB, Yuen TG, et al. Histologic and physiologic evaluation of electrically stimulated peripheral nerve: considerations for the selection of parameters. Ann Biomed Eng 1989;17(1):39–60.
6. Tyler DJ, Durand DM. Functionally selective peripheral nerve stimulation with a flat interface nerve electrode. IEEE Trans Neural Syst Rehabil Eng 2002;10: 294–303.
7. Tyler DJ, Durand DM. A slowly penetrating interfascicular nerve electrode for selective activation of peripheral nerves. IEEE Trans Rehabil Eng 1997;5(1):51–61.
8. Bamford JA, Mushahwar VK. Intraspinal microstimulation for the recovery of function following spinal cord injury. Prog Brain Res 2011;194:227–39.
9. Agarwal S, Triolo RJ, Kobetic R, et al. Long-term user perceptions of an implanted neuroprosthesis for exercise, standing, and transfers after spinal cord injury. J Rehabil Res Dev 2003;40(3):241–52.
10. Cogan SF. Neural stimulation and recording electrodes. Annu Rev Biomed Eng 2008;10(1):275–309.
11. Geddes LA, Roeder R. Criteria for the selection of materials for implanted electrodes. Ann Biomed Eng 2003;31(7):879–90.
12. Prasad A, Sanchez JC. Quantifying long-term microelectrode array functionality using chronic in vivo impedance testing. J Neural Eng 2012;9(2):026028.
13. Khaled I, Cheng C, Elmallah S, et al. A flexible base electrode array for intraspinal microstimulation. IEEE Trans Biomed Eng 2013;60:2904–13.
14. Grill WM, Norman SE, Bellamkonda RV. Implanted neural interfaces: biochallenges and engineered solutions. Annu Rev Biomed Eng 2009;11:1–24.
15. Anderson K. Targeting recovery: priorities of the spinal cord injured population. J Neurotrauma 2004;21(10):1371–83.
16. Keith MW, Kilgore KL, Peckham PH, et al. Tendon transfers and functional electrical stimulation for reconstruction of hand function in spinal cord injury. J Hand Surg Am 1996;21:89–99.
17. Chae J, Kilgore KL, Triolo RJ, et al. Functional neuromuscular stimulation in spinal cord injury. Phys Med Rehabil Clin N Am 2000;11(1):209–26.
18. Scott TR, Haugland M. Command and control interfaces for advanced neuroprosthetic applications. Neuromodulation 2001;4(4):165–75.
19. Nathan RH. Functional electrical stimulation of the upper limb: charting the forearm surface. Med Biol Eng Comput 1979;17(6):729–36.
20. Popovic M, Popovic D, Keller T. Neuroprostheses for grasping. Neurol Res 2002;24:443–52.

21. Popovic R, Thrasher T, Adams M, et al. Functional electrical therapy: retraining grasping in spinal cord injury. Spinal Cord 2006;44(3):143–51.

22. Peckham PH, Keith MW, Kilgore KL, et al. Efficacy of an implanted neuroprosthesis for restoring hand grasp in tetraplegia: a multicenter study. Arch Phys Med Rehabil 2001;82:1380–8.

23. Wuolle KS, Van Doren CL, Bryden AM, et al. Satisfaction and usage of a hand neuroprosthesis. Arch Phys Med Rehabil 1999;80:206–13.

24. Taylor P, Esnouf J, Hobby J. The functional impact of the Freehand system on tetraplegic hand function, clinical results. Spinal Cord 2002;40:560–6.

25. Kilgore KL, Hoyen HA, Bryden AM, et al. An implanted upper extremity neuroprosthesis utilizing myoelectric control. J Hand Surg Am 2008;33:539–50.

26. Hart RL, Bhadra N, Montague FW, et al. Design and testing of an advanced implantable neuroprosthesis with myoelectric control. IEEE Trans Neural Syst Rehabil Eng 2011;19(1):45–53.

27. Peckham PH, Kilgore KL. Challenges and opportunities in restoring function after paralysis. IEEE Trans Biomed Eng 2013;60(3):602–9.

28. Moss CW, Kilgore KL, Peckham PH. A novel command signal for motor neuroprosthetic control. Neurorehabil Neural Repair 2011;25(9):847–54.

29. Donoghue JP, Nurmikko A, Black M, et al. Assistive technology and robotic control using motor cortex ensemble-based neural interface systems in humans with tetraplegia. J Physiol 2007;579(Pt 3):603–11.

30. Williams MR, Kirsch RF. Evaluation of head orientation and neck muscle EMG signals as command inputs to a human-computer interface for individuals with high tetraplegia. IEEE Trans Neural Syst Rehabil Eng 2008;16(5):485–96.

31. Rohde L, Bonder B, Triolo R. An exploratory study of perceived quality of life with implanted standing neuroprostheses. J Rehabil Res Dev 2012;49(2):265–78.

32. Creasey GH, Ho CH, Triolo RJ, et al. Clinical applications of electrical stimulation after spinal cord injury. J Spinal Cord Med 2004;27:365–75.

33. Triolo RJ, Bailey SN, Miller ME, et al. Longitudinal performance of a surgically implanted neuroprosthesis for lower extremity exercise, standing, and transfers after spinal cord injury. Arch Phys Med Rehabil 2012;93(5):896–904. http://dx.doi.org/10.1016/J.APMR.2012.01.001.

34. Nataraj R, Audu M, Triolo R. Comparing joint kinematics and center of mass acceleration for feedback control of standing by functional neuromuscular stimulation. J Neuroeng Rehabil 2012;9:25. http://dx.doi.org/10.1186/1743-0003-9-25.

35. Mushahwar VK, Jacobs PL, Normann RA, et al. New functional electrical stimulation approaches to standing and walking. J Neural Eng 2007;4:S181–97.

36. Kobetic R, Triolo RJ, Uhlir J, et al. Implanted functional electrical stimulation system for mobility in paraplegia: a follow-up case report. IEEE Trans Rehabil Eng 1999;7(4):390–8.

37. Cikajlo I, Matjacic Z, Bajd T, et al. Sensory supported FES control in gait training of incomplete spinal cord injury persons. Artif Organs 2005;29(6):459–61.

38. Hardin E, Kobetic R, Murray L, et al. Walking after incomplete spinal cord injury with an implanted FES system. J Rehabil Res Dev 2007;44(3):333–46.

39. Bailey SN, Hardin E, Kobetic R, et al. Neuroprosthetic and neurotherapeutic effects of implanted electrical stimulation for ambulation after incomplete spinal cord injury. J Rehabil Res Dev 2010;47(1):7–16.

40. Dutta A, Kobetic R, Triolo R. Gait initiation with electromyographically triggered electrical stimulation in people with partial paralysis. J Biomech Eng 2009;131(8):081002. http://dx.doi.org/10.1115/1.3086356.

41. Hettinga DM, Andrews BJ. Oxygen consumption during functional electrical stimulation-assisted exercise in persons with spinal cord injury: implications for fitness and health. Sports Med 2008;38(10):825–38.

42. Sadowsky CL, Hammond ER, Strohl AB, et al. Lower extremity functional electrical stimulation cycling promotes physical and functional recovery in chronic spinal cord injury. J Spinal Cord Med 2013;36(6):623–31. http://dx.doi.org/10.1179/2045772313Y.0000000101.

43. Dutta A, Kobetic R, Triolo R. Ambulation after incomplete spinal cord injury with EMG-triggered functional electrical stimulation. IEEE Trans Biomed Eng 2008;55(2):791–4.

44. Fisher L, Miller M, Nogan S, et al. Standing after spinal cord injury with four contact nerve-cuff electrodes for quadriceps stimulation. IEEE Trans Neural Syst Rehabil Eng 2008;16(5):473–8. http://dx.doi.org/10.1109/TNSRE.2008.2003390.

45. Fisher L, Tyler D, Triolo R. Optimization of selective stimulation parameters for multi-contact electrodes. J Neuroeng Rehabil 2013;10:25. http://dx.doi.org/10.1186/1743-0003-10-25.

46. Audu M, Nataraj R, Gartman S, et al. Posture shifting after spinal cord injury using functional neuromuscular stimulation – a computer simulation study. J Biomech 2011;44:1639–45. http://dx.doi.org/10.1016/j.jbiomech.2010.12.020.

47. Kobetic R, To C, Schnellenberger J, et al. Development of a hybrid orthosis for standing, walking and stair climbing after spinal cord injury. J Rehabil Res Dev 2009;46(3):447–62.

48. Kukke SN, Triolo RJ. The effects of trunk stimulation on bimanual seated workspace. IEEE Trans Neural Syst Rehabil Eng 2004;12:177–85.

49. Spungen AM, Adkins RH, Steward CA, et al. Factors influencing body composition in persons with spinal cord injury: a cross-sectional study. J Appl Physiol (1985) 2003;95:2398–407.

50. Potten YJ, Seelen HA, Drukker J, et al. Postural muscle responses in the spinal cord injured persons during forward reaching. Ergonomics 1999;42:1200–15.

51. Hart N, Laffont I, de La Sota A, et al. Respiratory effects of combined truncal and abdominal support in patients with spinal cord injury. Arch Phys Med Rehabil 2005;86:1447–51.

52. Hobson DA, Tooms RE. Seated lumbar/pelvic alignment. A comparison between spinal cord-injured and noninjured groups. Spine 1992;17:293–8.

53. Curtis KA, Kindlin CM, Reich KM, et al. Functional reach in wheelchair users: the effects of trunk and lower extremity stabilization. Arch Phys Med Rehabil 1995;76:360–7.

54. Ueyoshi A, Shima Y. Studies on spinal braces. With special reference to the effects of increased abdominal pressure. Int Orthop 1985;9:255–8.

55. Wu GA, Lombardo LM, Triolo RJ, et al. The effects of combined trunk and gluteal neuromuscular electrical stimulation on posture and tissue health in spinal cord injury. PM R 2013;5:688–96.

56. Triolo RJ, Bailey SN, Miller ME, et al. Effects of stimulating hip and trunk muscles on seated stability, posture, and reach after spinal cord injury. Arch Phys Med Rehabil 2013;94:1766–75.

57. Triolo RJ, Bailey SN, Lombardo LM, et al. Effects of intramuscular trunk stimulation on manual wheelchair propulsion mechanics in 6 subjects with spinal cord injury. Arch Phys Med Rehabil 2013;94:1997–2005.

58. Davis JA, Triolo RJ, Uhlir JP, et al. Surgical technique for installing an 8-channel neuroprosthesis for standing. Clin Orthop Relat Res 2001;4:237–52.

59. Vette AH, Yoshida T, Thrasher TA, et al. A comprehensive three-dimensional dynamic model of the human head and trunk for estimating lumbar and cervical joint torques and forces from upper body kinematics. Med Eng Phys 2012; 34(5):640–9.

60. Murphy JO, Audu ML, Lombardo LM, et al. Feasibility of a closed-loop controller for righting seated posture after spinal cord injury. J Rehabil Res Dev 2014, in press.

61. Markova A, Mostow EN. US skin disease assessment: ulcer and wound care. Dermatol Clin 2012;30(1):107–11, ix.

62. Lyder CH, Wang Y, Metersky M, et al. Hospital-acquired pressure ulcers: results from the national Medicare Patient Safety Monitoring System study. J Am Geriatr Soc 2012;60:1603–8.

63. VanGilder C, MacFarlane GD, Harrison P, et al. The demographics of suspected deep tissue injury in the United States: an analysis of the International Pressure Ulcer Prevalence Survey 2006-2009. Adv Skin Wound Care 2010;23:254–61.

64. Mushahwar VK, Solis L. Mitigation of pressure ulcers using electrical stimulation. US patent application 12/362,725, Jan 2009.

65. Solis LR, Gyawali S, Seres P, et al. Effects of intermittent electrical stimulation on superficial pressure, tissue oxygenation, and discomfort levels for the prevention of deep tissue injury. Ann Biomed Eng 2011;39:649–63.

66. Gyawali S, Solis L, Chong SL, et al. Intermittent electrical stimulation redistributes pressure and promotes tissue oxygenation in loaded muscles of individuals with spinal cord injury. J Appl Physiol (1985) 2011;110:246–55.

67. Solis LR, Liggins A, Uwiera RR, et al. Distribution of internal pressure around bony prominences: implications to deep tissue injury and effectiveness of intermittent electrical stimulation. Ann Biomed Eng 2012;40(8):1740–59. http://dx.doi.org/10.1007/s10439-012-0529-0.

68. Solis LR, Twist E, Seres P, et al. Prevention of deep tissue injury through muscle contractions induced by intermittent electrical stimulation after spinal cord injury in pigs. J Appl Physiol (1985) 2013;114(2):286–96. http://dx.doi.org/10.1152/japplphysiol.00257.2012.

69. Bogie KM, Wang X, Triolo RJ. Long term prevention of pressure ulcers in high risk individuals: a single case study of the use of gluteal neuromuscular electrical stimulation. Arch Phys Med Rehabil 2006;87(4):585–91.

70. Bogie KM, Triolo RJ. The effects of regular use of neuromuscular electrical stimulation on tissue health. J Rehabil Res Dev 2003;40(6):469–75.

71. Bogie K, Ho CH, Chae J, et al. Dynamic therapeutic neuromuscular electrical stimulation for pressure relief. Am J Phys Med Rehabil 2004;83(3):240.

72. Mushahwar VK, Isaacson G, Ahmetovic A, et al. Apparatus and method for electrically stimulating pressure-loaded muscles. WIPO application WO 2013/113099 A1, January 2013.

73. Gaunt RA, Prochazka A. Control of urinary bladder function with devices: successes and failures. Prog Brain Res 2006;152:163–94.

74. Brindley GS. An implant to empty the bladder or close the urethra. J Neurol Neurosurg Psychiatry 1977;40:358–69.

75. Creasey GH, Dahlberg JE. Economic consequences of an implanted neuroprosthesis for bladder and bowel management. Arch Phys Med Rehabil 2001; 82(11):1520–5.

76. Sanders PM, Ijzerman MJ, Roach MJ, et al. Patient preferences for next generation neural prostheses to restore bladder function. Spinal Cord 2011;49(1):113–9.

77. Farag FF, Martens FM, Rijkhoff NJ, et al. Dorsal genital nerve stimulation in patients with detrusor overactivity: a systematic review. Curr Urol Rep 2012;13(5):385–8.

78. Lee YH, Kim SH, Kim JM, et al. The effect of semiconditional dorsal penile nerve electrical stimulation on capacity and compliance of the bladder with deformity in spinal cord injury patients: a pilot study. Spinal Cord 2012;50(4):289–93.

79. Possover M, Schurch B, Henle KP. New strategies of pelvic nerves stimulation for recovery of pelvic visceral functions and locomotion in paraplegics. Neurourol Urodyn 2010;29(8):1433–8.

80. Kirkham AP, Knight SL, Craggs MD, et al. Neuromodulation through sacral nerve roots 2 to 4 with a Finetech-Brindley sacral posterior and anterior root stimulator. Spinal Cord 2002;40(6):272–81.

81. Yoo PB, Horvath EE, Amundsen CL, et al. Multiple pudendal sensory pathways reflexly modulate bladder and urethral activity in patients with spinal cord injury. J Urol 2011;185(2):737–43.

82. McCoin JL, Bhadra N, Gustafson KJ. Electrical stimulation of sacral dermatomes can suppress aberrant urethral reflexes in felines with chronic spinal cord injury. Neurourol Urodyn 2013;32(1):92–7.

83. Boger AS, Bhadra N, Gustafson KJ. High frequency sacral root nerve block allows bladder voiding. Neurourol Urodyn 2012;31(5):677–82.

84. Mushahwar VK, Horch KW. Proposed Specifications for a Lumbar Spinal Cord Electrode Array for Control of Lower Extremities in Paraplegia. IEEE Trans Rehabil Eng 1997;5:237–43.

85. Mushahwar VK, Horch KW. Selective Activation of Muscles in the Feline Hindlimb through Electrical Microstimulation of the Ventral Lumbo-Sacral Spinal Cord. IEEE Trans Rehabil Eng 2000;8(1):11–21.

86. Mushahwar VK, Horch KW. Muscle Recruitment through Electrical Stimulation of the Lumbo-sacral Spinal Cord. IEEE Trans Rehabil Eng 2000;8(1):22–9.

87. Mushahwar VK, Collins DK, Prochazka A. Spinal Cord Microstimulation Generates Functional Movements in Chronically Implanted Cats. Exp Neurol 2000; 163(2):422–9.

88. Prochazka A, Mushahwar VK, McCreery D. Neural Prostheses: Pros and Cons. J Physiol (London) 2001;533:99–109.

89. Mushahwar VK, Horch KW. Selective Activation and Graded Recruitment of Functional Muscle Groups through Spinal Cord Stimulation. Ann N Y Acad Sci 1998;860:531–5.

90. Bamford J, Putman CT, Mushahwar VK. Intraspinal Microstimulation Preferentially Recruits Fatigue-Resistant Muscle Fibres and Generates Gradual Force in Rat. J Physiol (London) 2005;569.3:873–84.

91. Bamford JA, Todd KG, Mushahwar VK. The Effects of Intraspinal Microstimulation on Spinal Cord Tissue in the Rat. Biomaterials 2010;31:5552–63.

92. Lau B, Guevremont L, Mushahwar VK. Open- and Closed-loop Control Strategies for Restoring Standing using Intramuscular and Intraspinal Stimulation. IEEE Trans Neural Syst Rehabil Eng 2007;15:273–85.

93. Saigal R, Renzi CG, Mushahwar VK. Intraspinal Microstimulation Generates Functional Limb Movements after Spinal Cord Injury. IEEE Trans Neural Syst Rehabil Eng 2004;12:430–40.

94. Holinski BJ, Mazurek KA, Everaert DG, et al. Restoring stepping after spinal cord injury using intraspinal microstimulation and novel control strategies. Conf Proc IEEE Eng Med Biol Soc 2011;2011:5798–801. http://dx.doi.org/10.1109/IEMBS.2011.6091435.

95. Mazurek K, Holinski BJ, Everaert DG, et al. Feedforward and Feedback Control for Over-ground Locomotion in Anesthetized Cats. J Neural Eng 2012;9(2):026003.

96. Guevremont L, Norton JA, Mushahwar VK. A Physiologically-based Controller for Generating Overground Locomotion using Functional Electrical Stimulation. J Neurophysiol 2007;97:2499–510.
97. Federici T, Hurtig CV, Burks KL, et al. Surgical technique for spinal cord delivery of therapies: demonstration of procedure in gottingen minipigs. J Vis Exp 2012;(70):e4371.
98. Riley J, Federici T, Polak M, et al. Intraspinal stem cell transplantation in amyotrophic lateral sclerosis: a phase I safety trial, technical note, and lumbar safety outcomes. Neurosurgery 2012;71(2):405–16. http://dx.doi.org/10.1227/NEU.0b013e31825ca05f [discussion: 416].

Spasticity and the Use of Intrathecal Baclofen in Patients with Spinal Cord Injury

CrossMark

Seema R. Khurana, DO[a],*, Deep S. Garg, MD[b]

KEYWORDS

• Baclofen • Spasticity • Spasms • Tone

KEY POINTS

- Spasticity and spasms are serious complications for many patients with spinal cord injury (SCI), as they both indicate an imbalance in the mechanisms that regulate reflex motor activity at the level of the spinal cord.
- Muscle spasms and spasticity constitute a significant problem, interfering with rehabilitation and leading to impairments in quality of life in addition to medical complications.
- Intrathecal baclofen (ITB) may be an effective option to consider in patients who cannot tolerate the adverse effects of high-dose oral baclofen.
- ITB administration is indicated when spasticity continues to produce a clinical disability despite trials of oral treatments and other alternatives in patients who have functional goals and/or pain without contractures.
- Intrathecal administration achieves high concentrations of the drug in the spinal cord with small dosages, thus reducing the incidence of central nervous system side effects. In addition, it allows for flexible dosing patterns to suit an individual patient's lifestyle.
- The 2 major risks of ITB involve symptoms related to overdose or withdrawal; the latter is more important because of the associated severe effects on clinical status and the possibility of death, but is responsive to rapid treatment.
- Severe spasticity of spinal origin has been shown to respond dramatically to the long-term intrathecal administration of baclofen when it is used in appropriate patients with spasticity.

INTRODUCTION

Chronic, intractable spasticity is a major health problem for patients with spinal cord injury (SCI), and can cause significant disability and impairments in quality of life.[1–3] Undesired muscle spasms and increased motor tone often make activities of daily

[a] Department of Physical Medicine and Rehabilitation, University of Miami, Miller School of Medicine, 1120 Northwest 14th Street, CRB Room 948, Miami, FL 33136, USA; [b] Department of Physical Medicine and Rehabilitation, Jackson Memorial Hospital, University of Miami-Miller School of Medicine, Miami, FL, USA
* Corresponding author.
E-mail address: skhurana@med.miami.edu

Phys Med Rehabil Clin N Am 25 (2014) 655–669
http://dx.doi.org/10.1016/j.pmr.2014.04.008
1047-9651/14/$ – see front matter © 2014 Elsevier Inc. All rights reserved.

living, transfers, self-care, and even sitting comfortably difficult or near impossible for patients with both complete and incomplete lesions.[3] Using a database of self-reported secondary medical problems in recently injured SCI patients, 53% reported spasticity as the most disabling complication, followed by pain and pressure ulcers. In a survey of 500 long-standing SCI patients, spasticity was the second most reported complication after urinary tract infections, and was found to occur much more frequently in SCI with Frankel grades of B or C, and more so in incomplete tetraplegics than in paraplegics.[4]

Baclofen, the administration of which is primarily indicated for the spasticity of spinal origin, was first introduced for clinical use in Europe in the 1960s.[2] Although oral baclofen continues to be used successfully to treat spasticity, when given intrathecally it has a more potent effect, requiring approximately one-hundredth of the oral dose, although this ratio varies greatly among patients. The development of implantable pump and catheter drug-delivery systems has allowed for the continuous infusion of baclofen into the intrathecal space, and remains an effective method of controlling rigidity and spasticity of spinal origin in appropriately selected patients.[5]

DEFINITION OF SPASTICITY AND SPASMS

Spasticity is a state of sustained, increased muscle contractility that can occur in many diseases of central origin such as stroke, cerebral palsy, multiple sclerosis, and amyotrophic lateral sclerosis. Clinically it is defined as a motor disorder characterized by a velocity-dependent increase in tonic stretch reflexes with exaggerated tendon jerks, resulting from hyperexcitability of the stretch reflex, as one component of the upper motor neuron syndrome.[6] It is a combination of clinical signs characterized by increased muscle tone with or without the presence of clonus and muscle spasms, abnormal spinal reflexes, and increased resistance to passive movement.[1]

Muscle spasms are episodes of involuntary motor contractions that occur following a lesion of the ascending motor pathway.[1] These spasms are often painful, and can lead to serious complications such as decubitus ulcers, falls and fractures, and respiratory compromise.

The original Ashworth scale, which is referred to in many clinical studies (**Table 1**), is a simple 5-point Likert scale in which the observer's subjective opinion of the patient's resting muscle tone ranges from "normal" at the lowest grade to "rigid" at the highest. This original scale was revised to form the modified Ashworth scale (**Table 2**), which is the one most commonly used today in the clinical setting, by adjusting the lowest number from 0 to 1 and the highest from 4 to 5. There was also the addition of a category between 1 and 2, with 1 indicating a "catch" at the joint's end range of

Table 1 The Ashworth scale	
Score	Definition
0	No increase in muscle tone
1	Slight increase in muscle tone, manifested by a catch and release
2	More marked increase in muscle tone through most of the range of motion, but affected limb is easily moved
3	Considerable increase in muscle tone; passive movement difficult
4	Limb rigid in flexion or extension

Adapted from Braddom R, Nance P, Satkunam L, et al. Physical medicine and rehabilitation. 4th edition. Philadelphia: W.B. Saunders Company; 2011. p. 642–55; with permission.

Table 2
The modified Ashworth scale

Score	Definition
0	No increase in tone
1	Slight increase in muscle tone, manifested by a catch and release, or by minimal resistance at the end of the range of motion (ROM) when the affected part(s) is moved into flexion and extension
1+	Slight increase in muscle tone, manifested by a catheter, followed by minimal resistance throughout the remainder (less than half) of the ROM
2	More marked increase in muscle tone through most of the ROM, but affected part(s) easily moved
3	Considerable increase in muscle tone, passive movement difficult
4	Affected part(s) rigid in flexion or extension

Adapted from Bohannon RW, Smith MB. Interrater reliability of a modified Ashworth scale of muscle spasticity. Phys Ther 1987;67(2):206–7; and Penn RD, Savoy SM, Corcos D, et al. Intrathecal baclofen for severe spinal spasticity. N Engl J Med 1989;320:1517–54, with permission.

motion and 1+ indicating a "catch" closer to the midpoint of the joint's range of motion.[7]

Another method of assessing spasticity is the Penn Spasm Frequency score (**Table 3**), which is an ordinal ranking of the patient-reported frequency of leg spasms per day and per hour. A major limitation of this is that the frequency of spasms can be affected by activity level, and it does not take into account the length of each spasm.

THE INCIDENCE OF SPASTICITY IN SCI PATIENTS

Spasticity is a prevalent issue for patients with SCI, and becomes more so with increasing time after injury and resolution of spinal shock.[8] Problematic spasticity occurs in 40% to 60% of patients with SCI and multiple sclerosis, which results in a significant impact on activities of daily living and patient independence. Its treatment must be based on individualized clinical decisions by the physician in conjunction with the patient and family or caretaker.

Maynard and colleagues[8] reviewed 2 major epidemiologic studies in patients after traumatic SCI, exploring the incidence and severity of spasticity development in addition to the incidence of spasticity treatment among these patients. The investigators found that spasticity development and treatment are common but not inevitable sequelae of SCI, with the incidence of spasticity being higher among cervical and upper thoracic rather than lower thoracic and lumbosacral levels of injury. This finding

Table 3
Penn Spasm Frequency score

Score	Criteria
0	None
1	No spontaneous spasms; vigorous sensory and motor stimulation results in spasms
2	Occasional spontaneous spasms occurring less than once per hour
3	Greater than 1 but less than 10 spontaneous spasms per hour
4	Greater than 10 spontaneous spasms per hour

Adapted from Penn RD, Savoy SM, Corcos D, et al. Intrathecal baclofen for severe spinal spasticity. N Engl J Med 1989;320:1517–54; with permission.

may be due to primarily upper motor neuron damage to the spinal cord at the cervical and upper thoracic levels of injury, in contrast to lower motor neuron damage to the conus medullaris or cauda equina at the lower thoracic and lumbosacral levels. In addition, although the relationship between spasticity and level of injury must be taken into consideration, grouping patients by the presence of quadriplegia versus paraplegia is likely inappropriate. When investigating the incidence of and treatment of spasticity, multiple studies have found that spasticity is more common and more severe in patients with Frankel grade B and C lesions as opposed to grade A or D, and, by the same token, more common in patients with motor incomplete lesions than with motor complete lesions.

WHEN TO TREAT SPASTICITY

The first step in the management of all problematic spasticity is to identify, address, and treat any remediable causes and factors (ie, urinary tract infection [UTI], impacted stool, pressure sore, ingrown toenail, and so forth). If such measures are ineffective then it is appropriate to pursue treatment until a therapeutic response is obtained.[9]

The successful management of spasticity can be a therapeutic challenge, as its clinical presentation is highly variable among patients. Thus, the health care provider must assess each individual independently to determine whether spasticity is proving advantageous rather than disadvantageous.

To do this one must first establish whether there is a functional problem caused by the spasticity, and determine the related goals of treatment for the patient and/or caregiver. Despite common belief, the effects of spasticity might not always be negative. For example, spasticity can stabilize weakened legs, allowing a patient to stand or transfer and have improved bed mobility. Spasticity can also be a functionally helpful factor by being protective against skeletal muscle atrophy, indirectly aiding in functional independence and ambulation, and decreasing the incidence of fracture. Moreover, spasticity has been reported to increase glucose uptake and thereby reduce the risk for diabetes in those with SCI. The goal of functional improvement must therefore consider the balance of treatment effects.[9]

TREATMENT OPTIONS AVAILABLE FOR SPASTICITY

Various pharmacologic interventions are available to manage spasticity following SCI. The treatment approach to spasticity usually relies on a combination of physical modalities and therapies, such as stretching to promote relaxation, mechanical bracing, and the use of transcutaneous electrical nerve stimulation, in addition to medications used as monotherapy or in conjunction with the physical modalities.

Several oral agents are available that target increased muscle tone. A Cochrane systematic review was conducted to assess the effectiveness and safety of several drugs with antispastic effects, such as baclofen, dantrolene, tizanidine, gabapentin, clonidine, and diazepam, which are commonly used as a first-line treatment.[4] Of these drugs only dantrolene has a peripherally acting mechanism of action. Another peripherally acting, but longer-lasting, treatment option is botulinum toxin type A (Botox), which is used to treat focal spasticity or localized spasms.[10] Phenol is less commonly used nowadays, but when the patient reaches a maximum dose of Botox and still needs injections in other sites, it is considered.[10] The other drugs, which are primarily centrally acting, thus predispose to greater side effects. Adverse effects of baclofen (**Table 4**) appear to be dose related and usually appear at doses greater than 60 mg/d, with the rate of medication discontinuation ranging from between 4% and 27%.[11]

Table 4
Adverse effects of oral baclofen administration for treatment of spasticity based on meta-analysis of multiple prospective trials

Symptom	Range of Percentage of Patients Affected
Weakness	0.8–68.7
Somnolence	7–70
Vertigo	4.5–13
Headache	1.5–17
Nausea	1.7–24
Vomiting	2–10
Depression	2–19
Dry mouth	4.7–21.7
Bladder symptoms	7.6–11.5

Adapted from Dario A, Tomei G. A benefit-risk assessment of baclofen in severe spinal spasticity. Drug Saf 2004;27(11):799–818; with permission.

Studies have shown that patients with spasticity resulting from SCI generally tend to have a more favorable response to baclofen than those with spasticity of cerebral origin, with significant improvements seen with oral baclofen alone (**Table 5**).[1] Most patients with spasticity are generally treated according to a protocol whereby baclofen, with or without diazepam, is often the first step in management followed by other drugs such as tizanidine or Botox for localized symptoms. However, there is no unified supporting evidence for this commonly used therapeutic approach,[4] and often it is used at the sole discretion of the treating physician's experience and judgment.

INTRATHECAL BACLOFEN THERAPY

Continuous ITB infusion via a programmable pump was first introduced by Penn and Kroin in 1984 for the treatment of chronic, medically intractable spasticity of spinal origin.[12] Since its introduction, there have been several clinical reports on ITB indicating that it was very effective.[13] Between May 1988 and July 1990, a nationwide long-term multicenter study was conducted in the United States using a total of 93 patients, 59 of them with spasticity secondary to SCI, to evaluate whether ITB therapy could be a safe and effective long-term treatment of chronic intractable spasticity.[3] The investigators found that severe spasticity of spinal original responded "dramatically" to long-term administration of ITB. In addition, the ability of the pump to accommodate the lifestyle needs of various patient types (ie, with some preserved motor or

Table 5
Percentage of clinical improvement (CI) of spasticity in studies of oral baclofen in spinal cord injury

No. of Patients	% CI in Spasticity	% CI in Spasms	Duration of Study	Type of Trial
72	87	96	>6 y	Open-label
137	80	85		Open-label
11 (crossover)	55	72	4 wk	Placebo-controlled

Adapted from Dario A, Tomei G. A benefit-risk assessment of baclofen in severe spinal spasticity. Drug Saf 2004;27(11):799–818; with permission.

sensory function) with flexibility in drug dose rate and patterns was a significant advantage.[3] Since 1992, ITB therapy has been used in more than 60,000 people worldwide to manage severe spasticity related to a variety of conditions. Sampson and colleagues[14] estimated that approximately 5% to 10% of SCI patients will require intrathecal drug-delivery systems to treat excessive spasticity.[11]

Advantages of ITB Therapy

Baclofen, which is structurally similar to γ-aminobutyric acid (GABA), binds to GABA-B receptors in the central nervous system located within the brainstem and dorsal horn of the spinal cord. By suppressing the release of excitatory neurotransmitters involved in monosynaptic and polysynaptic reflexes, it reduces muscle tone and spasms.[3]

High doses of oral baclofen are often required to manage severe spasticity in SCI patients, especially as increasing time passes after injury and the dose requirements of the oral form continue to increase. Although it is a highly effective medication, large orally administered doses of baclofen can lead to well-known cerebral side effects such as drowsiness and confusion (see **Table 4**); this is due to its pharmacokinetics and systemic absorption, which allow only small concentrations of the drug to reach the spinal cord and cerebrospinal fluid (CSF) despite high oral doses. Thus, intrathecal administration of the same drug directly into the lumbar subarachnoid space at different spinal levels (selected based on symptoms) leads to the avoidance of cerebral side effects while allowing for a high concentration of it to diffuse into the superficial layers of the spinal cord dorsal horn.[3] Intrathecal baclofen exhibits selectivity for the spinal cord as the concentration of intrathecally injected baclofen diminishes in the cranial direction.[15]

A review of the literature shows that continuous ITB therapy causes a significant decrease in spasticity and spasms, as reported by changes on the Ashworth scale and Penn Spasm Frequency scale in most patients. Numerous clinical studies, including double-blind, placebo-controlled, open prospective uncontrolled trials, open-label longitudinal trials, and retrospective trials, have shown the average improvement in spasticity to be greater than 85%, with spasms reported to have been improved by approximately 66%.[2]

Although most available literature emphasizes evaluating the effects of ITB based on clinically relevant neurologic, neurophysiologic, and urologic outcome measures such as the Ashworth scale, spasm score, electromyography, or bladder function, there are also considerable data available on the beneficial effects of ITB on quality of life.[16–21] Middel and colleagues[16] conducted a randomized, double-blind, multicenter trial measuring health-related quality of life and health status measures in patients with chronic, disabling spasticity who had failed to respond to maximum doses of oral baclofen, dantrolene, and tizanidine. Using validated health status measures such as the sickness impact profile (SIP) and Hopkins symptom checklist (HSCL), they found substantial improvement in physical and mental health, mobility, and sleep and rest subscales on the SIP, and in the HSCL mental health scale in patients who underwent ITB therapy.[17]

The Appropriate Time when SCI Patients Should be Considered for ITB Therapy

Other options for management should be considered when spasticity begins to plateau despite optimum conservative management, which can include multiple oral agents for at least 6 weeks or a trial of Botox for localized cases. In a study reporting the incidence of spasticity 1 year after SCI, 67% of patients had developed spasticity associated with spasms, 37% had received antispastic medication, and 11% had failed to respond to treatment.[4]

Before initiating any invasive therapies, it is always important to rule out other causes of worsening or refractory spasticity in SCI, such as UTI or syrinx. It is also important to evaluate the patient and caretaker and determine whether they meet the cognitive, social, and physical demands required to maintain the pump, make follow-up appointments, keep track of side effects, and so forth. It is also understood that relative contraindications exist in patients on anticoagulant therapy with coagulation disorders, anatomic abnormality of the spine, and localized or systemic infection.[11]

Lastly, regardless of injury level or severity, the patient should have functional goals (which can include pain relief) that are anticipated to be met with improvement in spasticity. Common examples of spasticity-limited functional goals are to improve speed and safety of wheelchair transfers, improve the performance of activities of daily living such as dressing, and facilitate perineal hygiene by reducing thigh adductor or pectoral muscle spasticity, thus facilitating ease of caregiver assistance.[9] Even ambulatory patients, that is, those with an American Spinal Injury Association impairment classification of D, can be potential candidates for low-dose ITB therapy provided that an improvement in spasticity will cause change in function.

How to Determine Who is a Good Candidate for ITB

A screening test is generally performed after a thorough evaluation is completed and the provider thinks that the patient may be a good candidate for the trial. This procedure generally involves administering a bolus dose of baclofen via lumbar puncture or temporary catheter into the CSF under local anesthesia to screen for patient response to treatment.[11] Patients with scoliosis and fusions are candidates for the screening test, but the physician performing the trial should have experience with these patients, as such patients will also be more challenging with regard to placement of the catheter if they have a successful trial.

On the day of the trial the patient usually does not take antispasticity medications. The patient presents in the morning and, as long as there are no contraindications, such as skin breakdown in the area where the injection will be administered, infection, and blood thinner temporarily stopped, the physician proceeds with the trial. In an environment with equipment available for resuscitation, under radiologic guidance a bolus of medication is injected via a lumbar puncture (usually 50 μg, but depending on the patient can be as slow as 25 μg). The medication has an onset of action of 30 minutes to 1 hour. Then, depending on available resources, the physical therapist (ideally) or any trained individual can begin conducting the assessment at 1 hour, with a repeat at 2 hours, 4 hours, and 6 hours. If at 8 hours the patient continues to have relief then that should be the starting dose, but if the patient does not continue to have relief the starting dose can be increased to twice the bolus dose.

The assessment can vary but should include the modified Ashworth scale at every increment, along with the patient's and caregiver's subjective assessments.

If for some reason no response is seen, it is possible to repeat the injection at 100 μg. There must be at least 24 hours between trial doses. If this still does not provide a response yet the patient does have spasticity on examination, it is possible to place a catheter and titrate the dose, and follow for up to 24 hours. Another possibility, depending on the level of the spinal cord lesion, is injection of the medication at a higher level.

After the trial it is mandatory that the patient has a follow-up appointment within a week, to discuss the results with the managing physician and answer further questions. If the trial has been successful the patient can be scheduled for implantation. In general, patients with a 2-point or more decrease in their Ashworth or Penn Spasm scale (see **Tables 1** and **3**) for a period of 4 to 8 hours after the injection can be considered for pump implantation.[11]

Where is an ITB Pump and Catheter Implanted and How is the Size Chosen?

At present, there are 3 choices for pumps, 2 of which have been approved for use with intrathecal baclofen (**Table 6**), with the Medtronics pump generally being the most commonly used and longest studied.

ITB is delivered via a metallic pump, which stores and releases the prescribed/programmed amount of medication through the catheter directly into the CSF. The pump is placed subfascially, usually in the anterolateral aspect of the lower abdomen near the waistline, under general anesthesia, with the catheter routed to the appropriate spinal cord level by a neurosurgeon. This approach allows for easy access during subsequent follow-up appointments for pump refills, during which the pump reservoir can be refilled by percutaneous injection into the filling port in the center of the pump. During this straightforward outpatient procedure a physician can make adjustments in dose, rate, and timing using an external programmer. The pump can and should be replaced at the end of its battery life, after approximately 5 to 7 years.[11]

A recently developed catheter, the Ascenda intrathecal catheter (**Fig. 1**), is a 4-layer braided catheter that is 6 times stronger than previous catheters, and reduces problems such as kinks, breaks, and leaks.

It is important to assess where the patient's spasticity is occurring, whether in the lower extremities alone or in both upper and lower extremities. If it is in both the upper and lower extremities then one should attempt to place the catheter tip as high as T1; if the spasticity is only affecting the lower extremities, it can be placed between T6 and T10.

There are 2 different sizes of pump: 20 mL and 40 mL (**Figs. 2–4**). In general, most patients have the 40-mL pump unless the body size is small or the dose expected to be used is low. If the 40-mL pump is implanted it will allow for less frequent need for refills. However, it is important to keep in mind that the refill needs to occur based on

---

Table 6
Comparison of Medtronics SynchroMed II with Flowonix Medical Prometra and Codman & Shurleff MedStream

	Medications Approved for Infusion	Reservoir Volume	Drug Stability (d)	MRI
Medtronics[25]	Infumorph Prialt Intrathecal baclofen	20 mL/40 mL	180	1.5 T and 3.0 T; pump designed to restart after MRI
Flowonix[27]	Infumorph	20 mL	90	1.5 T but must empty and program pump to 0 mg/d before MRI (Flowonix Web site)
MedStream[26]	Intrathecal baclofen	20 mL/40 mL	120	3.0 T; but 50% failed to restart therapy after MRI (Shellock)

Comparing the pumps' peristaltic mechanism, the SynchroMed II can deliver up to 6 times the maximum dose and half the minimum dose of the MedStream.
Abbreviation: MRI, magnetic resonance imaging.

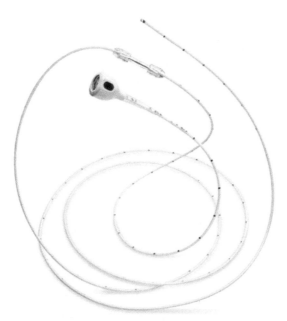

Fig. 1. Ascenda catheter. (*Courtesy of* Medtronic, Inc, Minneapolis, MN; with permission.)

drug stability. There are 2 baclofen formulations that the pump can be filled with, either Lioresal or Gablofen, which vary in both concentration and the type of packaging they arrive in (**Table 7**).

After the implantation of the pump it is important for the patient to be followed up on a weekly basis to have the dose titrated up; this has to be done gradually to prevent overdose, usually 10% per visit. Patients should remain on oral medications until their

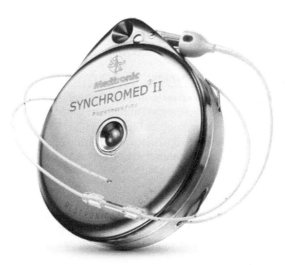

Fig. 2. A typical pump, such as this one manufactured by Medtronic, is a disc-shaped, titanium piece approximately 3 inches (7.6 cm) by 1 inch (2.5 cm) in size. (*Courtesy of* Medtronic, Inc, Minneapolis, MN; with permission.)

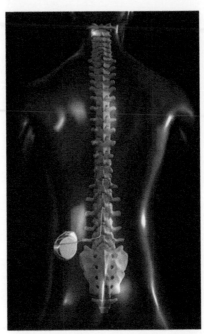

Fig. 3. The pump and catheter components of the intrathecal baclofen system are surgically implanted subcutaneously, below the fascia, in the anterolateral abdomen, usually in the lateral aspect of the lower abdominal wall. The catheter is then tunneled to the appropriate spinal level for continuous delivery of baclofen into the intrathecal space as per the dosing programmed onto the pump. (*Courtesy of* Medtronic, Inc, Minneapolis, MN; with permission.)

spasticity is controlled, then be slowly weaned off their oral medications. When patients are on a dose that controls their spasticity and are off their oral medications, they have the option to receive extra medications at different times during their day depending on their needs and lifestyle. This approach is referred to as flex dosing, in comparison with the original continuous dosing.

Risks and Adverse Effects of ITB Therapy

ITB pump malfunction can cause adverse effects in patients, such as fever, hallucinations, rebound spasticity, and even death (**Table 8**). It is important to rule out other potential causes of these symptoms, such as ulcers or UTI. If there is a problem with the pump-catheter system, it is important to identify the problem and address it because it can cause an incorrect amount of baclofen to be delivered. In some circumstances the baclofen cannot be delivered at all, causing severe withdrawal resembling neuroleptic malignant syndrome.

Catheter problems cause the most common complications, which include catheter-tip migration, dislocation, and dislodgment, and disconnection from the pump. Until recently, another common problem was breaking or kinking of the catheter. However, the introduction of a novel catheter in 2012 (Ascenda) has greatly diminished these problems.

Pump malfunction, which has been reported in up to 14% of patients, can also occur, and can result from rotor malfunction, reservoir depletion, programming/software malfunctions, and baclofen leakage from the pump.[22,23]

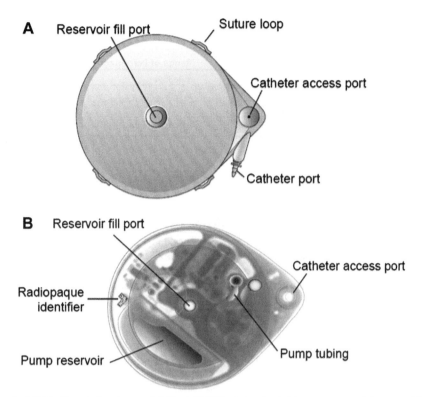

A Reservoir fill port   Suture loop

Catheter access port

Catheter port

B Reservoir fill port

Catheter access port

Radiopaque identifier

Pump reservoir   Pump tubing

Fig. 4. (A) Medtronic Synchromed II Model 8637, an implantable programmable pump. The catheter connects to the pump-catheter port. The pump is anchored in the pump pocket using the suture loops on the outside of the pump. (B) The drug is stored in the pump reservoir. As per a programmed prescription, the drug moves from the pump reservoir, through the pump tubing and catheter to the infusion site. The catheter access port (CAP) allows injection of baclofen directly into the implanted catheter for drug administration and diagnostic purposes. The CAP allows entry of a 24-gauge needle during refill procedures. (*Courtesy of* Medtronic, Inc, Minneapolis, MN; with permission.)

If a problem is suspected, it is suggested to first interrogate the pump and confirm the pump programming and reservoir status. One should then either obtain anteroposterior and lateral abdominal radiographs, which can help to visualize any catheter dislodgment or disconnection, or perform a catheter port aspiration to confirm that the catheter is properly connected and that CSF is able to be obtained.[24] If the problem is still not identified, a roller dye study can be performed whereby under fluoroscopy 2 to 3 mL of fluid is aspirated to prevent baclofen overdose, after which dye is injected into the accessory port and followed through the catheter to the intrathecal space.

Table 7 Comparison of Gablofen and Lioresal		
	Concentrations	**Packaging**
Gablofen	50, 500, 1000, and 2000 μg/mL	Prefilled syringes and ready-to-use vials
Lioresal	50, 500, and 2000 μg/mL	Glass ampules

Table 8
Adverse effects of intrathecal baclofen administration

Symptom	Range of Percentage of Patients Affected
Drowsiness	5.4–35.4
Nausea	0.7–4
Ejaculation impairment	0.8–1.5
Constipation	2.9–9.1

Other symptoms rarely seen were dizziness, blurred vision, slurred speech, confusion, and decreased memory.

Adapted from Dario A, Tomei G. A benefit-risk assessment of baclofen in severe spinal spasticity. Drug Saf 2004;27(11):799–818; with permission.

Special Considerations in Patients with an ITB Pump

1. If CSF is needed in a patient with an ITB pump, it is important to obtain it from the catheter access port and not in the traditional way, for 2 reasons: first, it is easy to obtain and second, it does not risk puncturing the catheter.
2. Patients on an ITB pump can undergo magnetic resonance imaging (MRI); however, depending on the pump there are certain protocols that must be followed. The most commonly used pump by Medtronics is safe at 1.5 T and 3 T, but following the MRI the patient is required to have the pump interrogated with the logs to ensure that the pump has restarted.
3. Patients with an ITB pump can travel, but it is important for them to always keep their most recent printout along with the medical ID card given to them at the time when the pump was implanted, thus allowing them to pass through security with fewer questions. Also, depending on how long they will be away, they should make sure that their refill date will not occur while away, and if so should receive a refill before they leave to prevent withdrawal from an empty pump.
4. The Medtronics pump can last a maximum of 7 years, with a usual pump life of 5 to 7 years. There is an elective replacement indicator (ERI) printed on every interrogation, which helps to determine how long before the pump needs to be replaced. When the ERI approaches the 12-month mark, it is important to start working with the patient to schedule replacement of the pump, because it can take some time for the patient to see the surgeon, receive authorization, and finally schedule a surgery date. If the pump and catheter are functioning well and there are no problems with the catheter, the pump will simply be replaced at the scheduled time.
5. If there are concerns about the pump not working or the physician would like to see whether bolus dosing would help, a bolus could be given at the beginning of the visit and monitored over 4 hours for improvement.

Future Directions

A research study is currently being conducted to evaluate the safety of Gablofen 3000 µg/mL. This study allows participants to use a higher concentration of Gablofen, which will allow less frequent pump refills. Because spasticity effects differ between patients and the response to treatment varies; both of these factors affect the daily dose of the medication required. The benefits of increasing the concentration of the medication are both social and economic. Socially, the patient's quality of life will improve because of fewer visits for refills, reduced cost of transportation to the facilities, and less time spent on these refills. Economically, fewer resources will be consumed in regard of personnel time and products used.

SUMMARY

Spasticity is a common complication and is a prevalent issue among patients with SCI. It can severely impair normal daily functions such as walking, eating, dressing, and even sitting comfortably, thus making it a significant contributing factor toward patient disability.[10] The overall evidence of efficacy of oral antispastic drugs in nonprogressive neurologic diseases such as SCI is weak and adverse drug reactions are common, as demonstrated by a systematic review of double-blind, randomized controlled trials conducted by Montane and colleagues.[10]

An evidence-based analysis of the effectiveness and cost-effectiveness of ITB for spasticity conducted by the Ontario Health Technology Assessment Series summarized their findings as level-2 evidence, supporting the effectiveness of ITB infusion for the short-term and long-term reduction of severe spasticity in patients who are unresponsive or cannot tolerate oral baclofen.[11]

Before considering invasive treatments for spasticity such as ITB, it is important to first confirm that all noninvasive treatment approaches, such as medications for generalized symptoms or Botox for localized symptoms, have been exhausted. The Cochrane review concluded that "the use of intrathecal baclofen should be restricted to true nonresponders" of other pharmacologic interventions "through a careful assessment of the nonresponse."[4]

After identifying a potential candidate for ITB therapy, including outlining specific functional goals, it becomes integral to confirm through the screening trial whether the patient would actually benefit from baclofen administered intrathecally. If this trial is successful, only then can the surgical process of pump implantation and dose titration occur.

It becomes the ethical and moral responsibility of the health care provider who recommends a patient for ITB therapy to ensure that such a patient is able to successfully adhere to a follow-up appointment schedule that involves dose adjustment via pump reprogramming and, even more importantly, refill of the pump with baclofen. Failure to do so for any reason can lead to serious side effects of withdrawal and even death, depending on the individual situation. When such an event does occur, several steps must be taken to ensure patient safety.

ITB, as with any implantable medical device that is manually programmed, does not come without its risks of infection, dislodgment or breakage of the catheter, pump dysfunction, and programming errors leading to underdosing or overdosing.

Several different kinds and sizes of pumps and catheter systems are available on the market today, along with different formulations of baclofen with varying concentrations to allow for optimal dosing schedules. There are also ongoing investigational studies aimed at further improving the physical system of the pump and catheter as well as the antispastic medication itself.

The goal of rehabilitation medicine is to provide optimal, individualized care to a patient that improves his or her functional abilities to their maximal capacity. For some patients ITB therapy may be the clinically appropriate option to allow them to reach their functional goals.

REFERENCES

1. Lewis K, Mueller W. Intrathecal baclofen for severe spasticity secondary to spinal cord injury. Ann Pharmacother 1993;27:767–74.
2. Dario A, Tomei G. A benefit-risk assessment of baclofen in severe spinal spasticity. Drug Saf 2004;27(11):799–818.

3. Coffey JR, Cahill D, Steers W, et al. Intrathecal baclofen for intractable spasticity of spinal origin: results of a long term multicenter study. J Neurosurg 1993;78:226–32.
4. Taricco M, Adone R, Pagliacci C, et al. Pharmacological interventions for spasticity following spinal cord injury. Cochrane Database Syst Rev 2000;(2):CD001131.
5. Nance P, Schryvers O, Schmidt B. Intrathecal baclofen therapy for adults with spinal spasticity: therapeutic efficacy and effect on hospital admissions. Can J Neurol Sci 1995;22:22–9.
6. American Academy of Neurology. Assessment: the clinical usefulness of botulinum toxin-A in treating neurologic disorders: report of the Therapeutics and Technology Assessment Subcommittee of the American Academy of Neurology. Neurology 1990;40:1332–6.
7. Bohannon RW, Smith MB. Interrater reliability of a modified Ashworth Scale of muscle spasticity. Phys Ther 1987;67(2):206–7.
8. Maynard FM, Karunas RS, Waring WP. Epidemiology of spasticity following traumatic spinal cord injury. Arch Phys Med Rehabil 1990;71:566–9.
9. Braddom R, Nance P, Satkunam L, et al. Physical medicine and rehabilitation. 4th edition. Philadelphia: W.B. Saunders Company; 2011. p. 642–55.
10. Montane E, Vallano A, Laporte JR. Oral antispastic drugs in nonprogressive neurologic diseases: a systematic review. Neurology 2004;63(8):1357–63.
11. Health Quality Ontario. Intrathecal baclofen pump for spasticity: an evidence-based analysis. Ont Health Technol Assess Ser 2005;5(7):1–93.
12. Plassat R, Perrouin VB, Menei P, et al. Treatment of spasticity with intrathecal Baclofen administration: long-term follow-up, review of 40 patients. Spinal Cord 2004; 42(12):686–93.
13. Zahavi A, Geertzen JH, Middel B, et al. Long term effect (more than five years) of intrathecal baclofen on impairment, disability, and quality of life in patients with severe spasticity of spinal origin. J Neurol Neurosurg Psychiatry 2004;75(11):1553–7.
14. Sampson FC, Hayward A, Evans G, et al. The effectiveness of intrathecal baclofen in the management of patients with severe spasticity. Sheffield (United Kingdom): Trent Institute for Health Services Research, Universities of Leicester, Nottingham and Sheffield; 2000.
15. Miracle AC, Fox MA, Ayyangar RN. Imaging evaluation of intrathecal baclofen pump-catheter systems. AJNR Am J Neuroradiol 2011;32:1158–64.
16. Middel B, Kuipers-Upmeijer H, Bouma J. Effect of intrathecal baclofen delivered by an implanted programmable pump on health related quality of life in patients with severe spasticity. J Neurol Neurosurg Psychiatry 1997;63:204–9.
17. Staal C, Arends A, Ho S. A self-report of quality of life of patients receiving intrathecal baclofen therapy. Rehabil Nurs 2003;28(5):159–63.
18. Sampson FC, Hayward A, Evans G, et al. Functional benefits and cost/benefit analysis of continuous intrathecal baclofen infusion for the management of severe spasticity. J Neurosurg 2002;96:1052–7.
19. Becker WJ, Harris CJ, Long ML. Long term intrathecal baclofen therapy in patients with intractable spasticity. Can J Neurol Sci 1995;22:208–17.
20. Postma TJ, Oenema D, Terpstra S, et al. Cost analysis of the treatment of severe spinal spasticity with a continuous intrathecal baclofen infusion system. Pharmacoeconomics 1999;15:395–404.
21. Ordia JI, Fischer E, Adamski E. Chronic intrathecal delivery of baclofen by a programmable pump for the treatment of severe spasticity. J Neurosurg 1996;85: 452–7.
22. Penn RD. Intrathecal baclofen for spasticity of spinal origin: seven years of experience. J Neurosur 1992;77:236–40.

23. Fluckiger B, Knecht H, Grossman S, et al. Device-related complications of long-term intrathecal drug therapy via implanted pumps. Spinal Cord 2008;46:639–43.
24. Miracle AC, Fox MA, Ayyangar RN, et al. Imaging Evaluation of Intrathecal Baclofen Pump-Catheter Systems. Am J Neurorad 2011;32:1158–64.
25. Medtronic data on file. 2012 Addendum to the Medtronic Neurosstimulation & Intrathecal Drug Delivery Systems Product Performance Report. 2013.
26. Shellock FG, Crivelli R, Venugopalan R. Programmable infusion pump and catheter:evaluation using 3-tesla magnetic resonance imaging. Neuromodulation 2008;11(3):163–70.
27. Flowonix Webiste. Prometra Programmable Pump System Brief summary. Available at: http://www.flowonix.com/. Accessed May 21, 2013.

Spinal Cord Injury Pressure Ulcer Treatment

An Experience-Based Approach

Gabriel Sunn, MD[a,b],*

KEYWORDS

- Pressure ulcer • Pressure ulcer treatment • Spinal cord injury • Wound dressing
- Wound healing

KEY POINTS

- Pressure ulcers must be adequately assessed to design proper treatment.
- Wound dressings should be designed based on depth and suspected wound biofilm.
- Pressure ulcers must be treated by offloading as a priority.
- Pressure ulcers must be adequately debrided of devitalized tissue.
- Negative-pressure wound therapy is the dressing of choice for most stage III and IV pressure ulcers.
- Surgical intervention must be considered when addressing a pressure ulcer.

Pressure ulcers are a major source of morbidity and mortality for spinal cord injury patients worldwide. Prevalence of pressure ulcers in persons with spinal cord injury has been shown to be up to 30% in patients with chronic spinal cord injury and up to 49% in patients in the acute rehabilitation phase.[1,2] A well-known complication of spinal cord injury is urinary tract infections. In Japan, pressure ulcers rival urinary tract infections in doubling the hospital length of stay and tripling medical expenses for patients with spinal cord injury.[3] In Canada the average monthly healthcare costs of a person with spinal cord injury living with a pressure ulcer in the community approach $5000.[4] Not only do pressure ulcers alter the lives of patients by increasing hospital length of stay and healthcare costs, but pressure ulcers can have a major impact on patients' lives in other ways. Depression is a known risk factor for developing a pressure ulcer, and hospitalization for a pressure ulcer in the patient with spinal cord injury and depression can lead to a suicide attempt.[5]

[a] Physical Medicine and Wound Rehabilitation, Spinal Cord Injury Unit, Miami VA Hospital, 1C, 1201 Northwest 16th Street, Miami, FL 33125, USA; [b] Department of Physical Medicine and Rehabilitation, Miller School of Medicine, University of Miami, PO Box 016960 (D-461), Miami, FL 33101, USA
* Physical Medicine and Wound Rehabilitation, Spinal Cord Injury Unit, Miami VA Hospital, 1C, 1201 Northwest 16th Street, Miami, FL 33125.
E-mail address: gabriel.sunn@gmail.com

Phys Med Rehabil Clin N Am 25 (2014) 671–680
http://dx.doi.org/10.1016/j.pmr.2014.05.002
1047-9651/14/$ – see front matter Published by Elsevier Inc.

pmr.theclinics.com

Classification of pressure ulcers is relatively straightforward and has been well-outlined by the National Pressure Ulcer Advisory Panel. The stages and categories discussed next can be found on the National Pressure Ulcer Advisory Panel Web site.

PRESSURE ULCER STAGES AND CATEGORIES
Category/Stage I: Nonblanchable Erythema

This stage includes intact skin with nonblanchable redness of a localized area usually over a bony prominence (**Table 1**). Darkly pigmented skin may not have visible blanching; its color may differ from the surrounding area. The area may be painful, firm, soft, warmer, or cooler compared with adjacent tissue. Category I may be difficult to detect in individuals with dark skin tones. It may indicate "at risk" persons.

Category/Stage II: Partial Thickness

This partial-thickness loss of dermis presents as a shallow open ulcer with a red-pink wound bed, without slough. It may also present as an intact or open or ruptured serum-filled or serosanginous-filled blister. It presents as a shiny or dry shallow ulcer without slough or bruising (bruising indicates deep-tissue injury). This category should not be used to describe skin tears, tape burns, incontinence-associated dermatitis, maceration, or excoriation.

Category/Stage III: Full-Thickness Skin Loss

This is full-thickness tissue loss. Subcutaneous fat may be visible but bone, tendon, or muscle is not exposed. Slough may be present but does not obscure the depth of tissue loss. It may include undermining and tunneling. The depth of a category/stage III pressure ulcer varies by anatomic location. The bridge of the nose, ear, occiput, and malleolus do not have (adipose) subcutaneous tissue and category/stage III ulcers can be shallow. In contrast, areas of significant adiposity can develop extremely deep category/stage III pressure ulcers. Bone or tendon is not visible or directly palpable.

Table 1
Pressure ulcer categories

Pressure Ulcer Category	Recommended Dressing	Trade Names
Stage I pressure ulcer	Offloading, noncontact/nonthermal ultrasound	Various specialty beds and mattresses, MIST
Stage II pressure ulcer	Collagenase, foam dressings, adherent dressings	Santyl, Polymem, Mepilex, Mefix, Medipore
Stage III pressure ulcer	Negative-pressure wound therapy, collagen dressings, skin substitutes	VAC, SNAP, Prisma, Fibracol, Dermagraft, Epifix, Amniofix, Matristem
Stage IV pressure ulcer	Negative-pressure wound therapy, collagen dressings, skin substitutes	VAC, SNAP, Prisma, Fibracol, Dermagraft, Epifix, Amniofix, Matristem
Unstageable pressure ulcer	Sharp debridement, cadexomer iodine dressings, silver dressings	Iodoflex, Silvasorb, Acticoat
Suspected deep tissue Injury	Offloading, noncontact/nonthermal ultrasound	Various specialty beds and mattresses, MIST

Category/Stage IV: Full-Thickness Tissue Loss

This includes full-thickness tissue loss with exposed bone, tendon, or muscle. Slough or eschar may be present. It often includes undermining and tunneling. The depth of a category/stage IV pressure ulcer varies by anatomic location. The bridge of the nose, ear, occiput, and malleolus do not have (adipose) subcutaneous tissue and these ulcers can be shallow. Category/stage IV ulcers can extend into muscle and/or supporting structures (eg, fascia, tendon, or joint capsule) making osteomyelitis or osteitis likely to occur. Exposed bone or muscle is visible or directly palpable.

ADDITIONAL CATEGORIES AND STAGES FOR THE UNITED STATES
Unstageable/Unclassified: Full-Thickness Skin or Tissue Loss, Depth Unknown

This includes full-thickness tissue loss in which actual depth of the ulcer is completely obscured by slough (yellow, tan, gray, green, or brown) and/or eschar (tan, brown, or black) in the wound bed. Until enough slough and/or eschar are removed to expose the base of the wound, the true depth cannot be determined; but it is either a category/stage III or IV. Stable (dry, adherent, intact without erythema or fluctuance) eschar on the heels serves as "the body's natural (biologic) cover" and should not be removed.

Suspected Deep Tissue Injury, Depth Unknown

This is characterized by purple or maroon localized areas of discolored intact skin or blood-filled blister caused by damage of underlying soft tissue from pressure and/or shear. The area may be preceded by tissue that is painful, firm, mushy, boggy, warmer, or cooler compared with adjacent tissue. Deep-tissue injury may be difficult to detect in individuals with dark skin tones. Evolution may include a thin blister over a dark wound bed. The wound may further evolve and become covered by thin eschar. Evolution may be rapid exposing additional layers of tissue even with optimal treatment.

DRESSING AND TREATMENT BY WOUND CLASSIFICATION

Treatments and pitfalls are outlined next according to pressure ulcer classification.

Stage I Pressure Ulcer

Stage I pressure ulcers are mainly characterized by nonblanchable erythema (**Figs. 1** and **2**). A key to distinguishing this type of ulceration is palpation, because this wound type cannot be accurately assessed by observation alone. An opportune time for skin assessment is in conjunction with nursing either on admission or during clinic visits to allow for dual examination. An appropriate algorithm for stage I pressure ulceration involves offloading and stimulation of local tissue area to prevent the wound from progressing. Unfortunately, most literature regarding offloading for wounds is based around diabetic foot ulcers. Prospective, randomized control studies examining effectiveness and outcomes of offloading strategies are warranted.[6] Offloading may be arranged according to developing wound location. Many inpatient offloading programs begin with bed rest, depending on the wound locations. Heels may be offloaded by placing pillows or foam devices to suspend the feet and prevent further bed contact. Ischial tuberosity pressure ulcers may be offloaded by placing the patient in bed and alternating lateral pillows to roll patient from side to side. Sacral injuries may be offloaded by preventing the head of the bed from being raised more than 30 degrees. Other less common ulcers may be offloaded by a variety of customized techniques focusing on preventing local contact with the surface while minimizing pressure

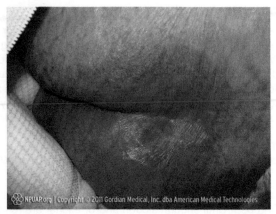

Fig. 1. Buttocks stage I pressure ulcer. (Used with permission of the National Pressure Ulcer Advisory. © NPUAP 2014.)

to the surrounding areas. Recommended devices include pillows and gel and foam pads. Although studies remain inconclusive, low-frequency noncontact nonthermal ultrasound may also be performed three to five times a week for 1 to 2 weeks to speed recovery of the injury. **Table 2** lists pressure ulcer locations and offloading techniques.

As with stage I pressure ulcers, suspected deep-tissue injuries must be immediately addressed with offloading and tracking as to the cause of the wound (**Figs. 3** and **4**). Wounds must be carefully monitored for progression or resolution. Noncontact nonthermal low-frequency ultrasound is highly recommended, for at least 5 days in a row, and has been found in our clinical experience to prevent progression of these wounds into open pressure ulcers.

Stage II Pressure Ulcer

One of the first determinations that must be made when examining a stage II pressure ulcer is that it is indeed a pressure ulcer (**Fig. 5**). As noted in the classification categories by the National Pressure Ulcer Advisory Panel, shallow ulcerations may be

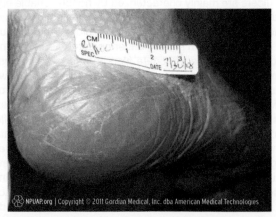

Fig. 2. Heel stage I pressure ulcer. (Used with permission of the National Pressure Ulcer Advisory. © NPUAP 2014.)

Table 2
Pressure ulcer locations and offloading techniques

Pressure Ulcer Location	Recommended Offloading Technique
Heel	Suspend feet by placing pillow under calf
Ischial tuberosity	Side lying of patient, head of bed no more than 30 degrees
Sacrum/coccyx	Side lying of patient, head of bed no more than 30 degrees

caused by moisture-related dermatitis or friction and trauma during transfers. This could easily confuse the treating physician, and although the wound may heal, it may recur if the inciting event is not identified. Chronic wounds are very likely to have developed biofilm.[7] An initial treatment of low-frequency noncontact, nonthermal ultrasound helps to destroy colonization by bacteria in the area. Alternatively, in a clinical setting where this treatment modality is unavailable, sharp curettage may provide removal of the biofilm, although without the additional benefits provided by ultrasound modality. After removal of biofilm, treatment dressings for stage II pressure ulcers are less complex than dressings for higher-stage ulcers.

It is important to note that surrounding skin must be prepared with cyanoacrolate before applying any dressing using adhesive. Dressings must also always be removed with adhesive remover. Countless hours of clinician time and effort are wasted if the surrounding skin is stripped of the necessary keratinocytes to heal the wound.

A typical dressing for a stage II pressure ulcer once the biofilm has been addressed is a daily or every other day dressing consisting of a thick layer of collagenase following a foam dressing, either thick or thin, followed by an adherent dressing. Because of the frequency of dressing changes for this type of wound, an adherent dressing with less aggressive adhesive should be chosen. When using collagenase, care must be taken not to use dressings or materials containing silver, because silver and other metal ions inactivate collagenase.[8]

Alternative dressings may be designed based on moisture of the wound. For a wound that is too wet, dry collagen dressings followed by dry hydrofiber dressing may be applied to absorb the excess exudate.

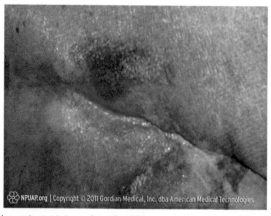

Fig. 3. Buttocks deep-tissue injury. (Used with permission of the National Pressure Ulcer Advisory. © NPUAP 2014.)

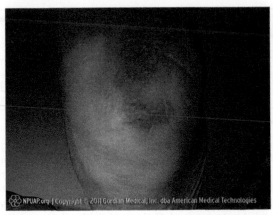

Fig. 4. Heel deep-tissue injury. (Used with permission of the National Pressure Ulcer Advisory. © NPUAP 2014.)

Stage III Pressure Ulcer

One of the first priorities when facing a stage III pressure ulcer is to remove any slough, or devitalized fat (**Fig. 6**). A practitioner must be familiarized with the various types of sharp debridement, which is best done clinically, the details of which are beyond the scope of this article. Common sharp debridement tools include curettes, scalpel, sharp scissors, and iris scissors. Once efforts have been made to ensure that all devitalized tissue has been removed, dressing options may be considered. For nearly all stage III pressure ulcers, negative-pressure wound therapy is the dressing of choice.[9] Depending on the size, location, depth, and drainage volume of the wound, a choice may be made between mechanical or electric-powered negative-pressure wound therapy. Smaller wounds with less drainage may be managed with a mechanically powered negative-pressure wound therapy device, changed twice weekly. Application of negative wound therapy devices is further delineated in the section regarding stage IV pressure ulcers.

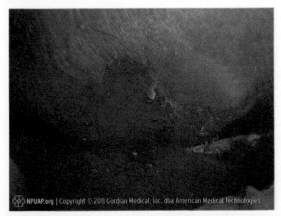

Fig. 5. Buttocks stage II pressure ulcer. (Used with permission of the National Pressure Ulcer Advisory. © NPUAP 2014.)

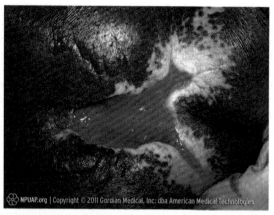

Fig. 6. Buttocks stage III pressure ulcer. (Used with permission of the National Pressure Ulcer Advisory. © NPUAP 2014.)

After an appropriate dressing has been selected for the stage III pressure ulcer, depth must be addressed as a priority. Adjunct dressings containing collagen, fibroblasts, or extracellular matrix may be placed into the wound depth to speed granulation. Care must be taken to use silicone contact layers to prevent adjunct dressings from being resorbed into the negative-pressure wound therapy devices. Once a wound has reached a superficial depth of 0.1 to 0.3 cm, dressings may be changed to be similar to those dressings used for stage II ulcers.

Stage IV Pressure Ulcer

As with stage III pressure ulcers, the first priority is to remove devitalized tissue including eschar (**Fig. 7**). If a deep wound causes high clinical suspicion for colonization, a beneficial dressing is one that contains cadexomer iodine, followed by hydrofiber to fill in depth and an adhesive dressing, changed daily or every other day.

Initial assessment of stage IV pressure ulcers must always include careful examination looking for exposed bone. If any suspicion exists for osteomyelitis, this must be excluded before progressing with wound treatment. Currently, magnetic resonance

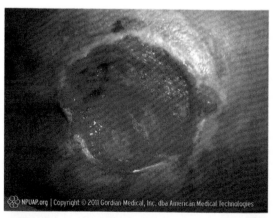

Fig. 7. Buttocks stage IV pressure ulcer. (Used with permission of the National Pressure Ulcer Advisory. © NPUAP 2014.)

imaging is the gold standard for diagnosis of osteomyelitis; however, some clinicians believe that if bone is visible or palpable in the wound, osteomyelitis may be presumed. If osteomyelitis is found, it must be treated simultaneously with the wound. Bone biopsy and culture may frequently be performed to allow for targeted antibiotic treatment.[10,11]

After a stage IV ulcer wound bed has been properly prepared by removing devitalized tissue and measures have been taken to reduce biofilm, a dressing should be designed, usually starting with a negative-pressure wound therapy device. Commonly, stage IV wounds exhibit tunnels and undermining that should be included in the dressing designs.

To correctly apply the negative-pressure therapy device, measures should be taken to ensure adequate sponge contact with all surfaces of the wound bed. Unless mechanical sponge debridement is desired, a silicone wound contact layer should be applied between all sponge layers and wound bed. As noted previously, surrounding skin should be carefully prepared before each dressing application with cyanoacrolate. Dressings should again also be removed with adhesive solvent to prevent stripping of adjacent keratinocytes.

As with stage III pressure ulcers, as soon as a dressing has been demonstrated as having reliable integrity with application and maintenance, consideration should be given toward adjunct dressings to speed the granulation process. In addition to dressings already mentioned, amniotic allografts may be used to fill in the defects. Negative-pressure wound therapy dressings may be changed once to twice per week. Once a stage IV pressure ulcer has become sufficiently superficial, finishing dressings may be applied as described in the section on stage II pressure ulcers.

Unstageable Pressure Ulcers

These wounds are necessarily addressed similarly to initial evaluation and treatment of stage IV pressure ulcers (**Fig. 8**). Initial dressing design may consist of cadexamer iodine dressings or heavily laden silver dressings to begin combating biofilm. These antimicrobial dressings may be followed by hydrofiber and adherent finishing dressings. These dressings may be changed daily along with serial sharp debridements to remove devitalized and necrotic tissue. Once a stage has been established for the wound, protocols as previously discussed may be followed.

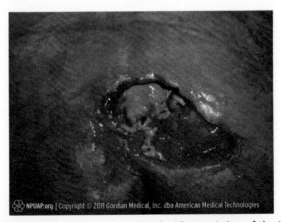

Fig. 8. Buttocks unstageable pressure ulcer. (Used with permission of the National Pressure Ulcer Advisory. © NPUAP 2014.)

SPECIAL CONSIDERATIONS

Tunneling is defined as a narrow tract extending from the wound bed and diving at an extended depth beyond the basic wound depth measurement. Tunnels must be regarded with high suspicion for foreign bodies and must be explored thoroughly. Hyperproliferative granulation tissue at the tunnel os or failure of the tunnel to resolve at a similar rate to the remainder of the wound can further provide evidence of a foreign body at the base of a tunnel. To address biofilm along the length of a tunnel, silver gel may be used along with the larger dressing. Silver nitrate applicator sticks are helpful not only in addressing the biofilm but also for probing depth of the tunnels.

Undermining is a separation of the wound bed often found underneath normal skin. Care should be taken when examining a wound to explore for tunneling and undermining. Interestingly, skin over undermining has been demonstrated to be normal. One method of approaching undermining is to place a layer of fibroblasts in the separation of the wound. Then, using negative-pressure wound therapy, a bolster is placed over the undermining allowing for some level of compression to augment attachment of the layers of dermis.

Much debate exists around where and when surgical intervention is merited. Current research is focused around establishing guidelines for surgical intervention for care of pressure ulcers. Clearly, a close working relationship with a surgeon is beneficial, because studies exist demonstrating that ulcer healing rates may be improved after surgical intervention.

The overriding conclusion for wound practice is that more research-based evidence is needed. A universally accepted standardized clinical management algorithm has yet to emerge. The available list of products to use on pressure ulcers is expansive and continues to grow on a daily basis, and a clinician must work diligently to maintain familiarity with treatment options including the evidence base behind them.

REFERENCES

1. Gélis A, Dupeyron A, Legros P, et al. Pressure ulcer risk factors in persons with spinal cord injury part 2: the chronic stage. Spinal Cord 2009;47(9):651–61.
2. Scheel-sailer A, Wyss A, Boldt C, et al. Prevalence, location, grade of pressure ulcers and association with specific patient characteristics in adult spinal cord injury patients during the hospital stay: a prospective cohort study. Spinal Cord 2013;51(11):828–33.
3. Kitagawa T, Kimura T. The influence of complications on rehabilitation of spinal cord injuries: economical minus effects and physical disadvantages caused by urinary tract infection and decubitus ulcer. J Nippon Med Sch 2002;69(3):268–77 [in Japanese].
4. Chan BC, Nanwa N, Mittmann N, et al. The average cost of pressure ulcer management in a community dwelling spinal cord injury population. Int Wound J 2013;10(4):431–40.
5. Dorsett P, Geraghty T. Health-related outcomes of people with spinal cord injury: a 10 year longitudinal study. Spinal Cord 2008;46(5):386–91.
6. Fowler E, Scott-Williams S, Mcguire JB. Practice recommendations for preventing heel pressure ulcers. Ostomy Wound Manage 2008;54(10):42–8, 50–2, 54–7.
7. James GA, Swogger E, Wolcott R, et al. Biofilms in chronic wounds. Wound Repair Regen 2008;16(1):37–44.
8. Shi L, Carson D. Collagenase Santyl ointment: a selective agent for wound debridement. J Wound Ostomy Continence Nurs 2009;36(Suppl 6):S12–6.

9. Ford CN, Reinhard ER, Yeh D, et al. Interim analysis of a prospective, randomized trial of vacuum-assisted closure versus the healthpoint system in the management of pressure ulcers. Ann Plast Surg 2002;49(1):55–61.

10. Pineda C, Espinosa R, Pena A. Radiographic imaging in osteomyelitis: the role of plain radiography, computed tomography, ultrasonography, magnetic resonance imaging, and scintigraphy. Semin Plast Surg 2009;23(2):80–9.

11. Srivastava A, Gupta A, Taly AB, et al. Surgical management of pressure ulcers during inpatient neurologic rehabilitation: outcomes for patients with spinal cord disease. J Spinal Cord Med 2009;32(2):125–31.

Dual Diagnosis
Traumatic Brain Injury with Spinal Cord Injury

David S. Kushner, MD*, Gemayaret Alvarez, MD

KEYWORDS

- Dual diagnosis • Traumatic brain injury • Spinal cord trauma • Diagnosis
- Prognosis • Complications • Rehabilitation

KEY POINTS

- Spinal cord injury (SCI) patients should be assessed for a co-occurring traumatic brain injury (TBI) on admission to a rehabilitation program.
- Incidence of a dual diagnosis may approach 60% with certain risk factors.
- The National Institute on Disability and Rehabilitation Research (NIDRR) SCI Model Systems started collecting data on co-occurring TBI in 2011 due to the high incidence of a dual diagnosis.
- Diagnosis of mild–moderate severity TBIs may be missed during acute care hospitalizations of SCI.
- Neuropsychological symptoms of a missed TBI diagnosis may be perceived during rehabilitation as noncompliance, inability to learn, maladaptive reactions to SCI, and poor motivation.
- There are life-threatening and/or quality-of-life–threatening complications of TBI that also may be missed if a dual diagnosis is not made.

INTRODUCTION

Rehabilitation strategies and expected outcomes for patients having a SCI can be complicated by a dual diagnosis of TBI. The reported incidence of concomitant brain and spinal cord injuries ranges from 25% to more than 60%, especially if the mechanism of injury was a motor vehicle collision or a fall.[1–5] Other factors that increase risk for a concomitant TBI are cervical level SCI, complete SCI level trauma, and initial trauma associated with alcohol intoxication.[3,4] The highest rate of concurrent TBI occurs in SCI patients with a C1 through C4 level of injury.[3]

Physical, cognitive, and/or emotional impairments that may result from a TBI pose important challenges in the rehabilitation of a dual diagnosis SCI patient. Physical

Department of Physical Medicine and Rehabilitation, University of Miami Miller School of Medicine, PO Box 016960 (D-461), Miami, FL 33101, USA
* Corresponding author.
E-mail address: dkushner@med.miami.edu

Phys Med Rehabil Clin N Am 25 (2014) 681–696
http://dx.doi.org/10.1016/j.pmr.2014.04.005
1047-9651/14/$ – see front matter © 2014 Elsevier Inc. All rights reserved.

impairments may include motor or sensory deficits. Motor impairments may involve deficits of strength, balance, and/or coordination. Sensory impairments may include deficits of touch or proprioception sensation and/or deficits of the special senses, such as vision. Cognitive impairments may include deficits of attention, information processing speed, problem solving, learning, memory, and communication. Emotional impairments may include apathy, emotional lability, agitation, aggression, disinhibition, impaired task initiation, anxiety, and depression.

The likelihood of significant physical, cognitive, and/or emotional impairments increases along the spectrum of worsening TBI severity from complicated mild TBI (MTBI) through moderate TBI to severe TBI. In SCI patients with a dual diagnosis of TBI, MTBI occurs most commonly and occurs in approximately 64% to 73% of cases whereas moderate TBI occurs in 10% to 23% and severe TBI in 17% to 23% of cases.[3,4] The relationship between SCI postrehabilitation functional outcomes and brain injury severities, however, is not necessarily linear,[6] although in general, as expected, the worst outcomes occur with a dual diagnosis of severe TBI. Also, the effect of severe TBI on motor recovery may be greatest in SCI patients having paraplegia rather than tetraplegia, probably due to a ceiling effect on motor recovery potential, although there are cognitive impairments that include memory and problem-solving deficits in both groups.[5] Paraplegic SCI patients with MTBI may have greater difficulties performing certain motor tasks, such as chair transfers, although cognitive deficits in uncomplicated MTBI tend to resolve prior to admission to inpatient rehabilitation.[5] Contusions involving motor brain areas resulting from moderate TBIs may result in contralateral motor deficits that exacerbate weakness resulting from an SCI. In experimental animal models, cortical contusions ipsilateral to a unilateral incomplete SCI at the C5 level enhanced forelimb motor recovery possibly due to the stimulation of plasticity in the contralateral motor cortex, which may have clinical relevance in patients having similar lesions.[1]

Prompt diagnosis of a concomitant TBI in an SCI patient is important for planning appropriate rehabilitation interventions to maximize functional returns and for the prevention, anticipation, and early treatment of possible related medical complications. A diagnosis of TBI, in particular mild and moderate severity TBIs, may be missed during the acute care hospitalization of an SCI patient, especially when there is a need for sedation, intubation, and/or the presence of acute trauma-related life-threatening issues. The symptoms, signs, and possible complications of a co-occurring TBI may not become evident until a patient is already admitted to an inpatient rehabilitation unit. Awareness on the part of the rehabilitation team regarding the potential for a dual diagnosis of TBI in traumatic SCI patients, as well as vigilance for related symptoms, signs, and/or complications, is important to improving both clinical and functional outcomes. Also, it is not uncommon for patients with a known diagnosis of co-occurring TBI with traumatic SCI to be assigned to a specialized TBI or SCI rehabilitation unit depending on which injury may be more severe.[1] Proper treatment and management strategies, however, are necessary for those patients who are admitted to rehabilitation with a known dual diagnosis of TBI/SCI regardless of whether they may be assigned to a TBI, an SCI, or a neurorehabilitation unit. TBI/SCI definition, diagnosis, pathologic features, evaluation, complications, and rehabilitation are discussed.

DEFINITION

A dual diagnosis of TBI with SCI occurs in patients having specific clinical and diagnostic features of both disorders resulting from trauma. The usual causes of the trauma are direct contact forces and/or rapid acceleration/deceleration movements resulting from assaults, crashes, and accidents involving motor vehicles, bicycles, pedestrians, construction, and sports.[7,8] The SCI may be defined as a traumatic lesion of the spinal cord or cauda equina, which may involve varying degrees of motor and/or sensory deficits.[4] SCI lesions may result in paraplegia or tetraplegia and may be classified as complete or incomplete per the American Spinal Injury Association impairment scale.[9] TBI may be defined as head trauma involving an alteration of consciousness having signs that may include confusion, loss of consciousness (LOC), and amnesia with or without other neurologic deficits.

Brain injury severity is classified as mild, moderate, or severe after a diagnosis is established based on criteria that may include initial Glasgow Coma Scale (GCS) scores, duration of posttraumatic amnesia (PTA), duration of LOC, and neuroimaging findings consistent with intracranial trauma, such as contusions, axonal shear injury, hemorrhages, and encephalomalacia.[3–5,7,8] GCS scores, PTA, LOC, and neuroimaging data are routinely collected by the NIDDR TBI Model System.[10] Standard classifications of TBI severity based on these 4 diagnostic criteria are provided in **Table 1**. Assessments of GCS scores, PTA durations, and LOC may be confounded, however, in SCI patients by hypoxia, intubation, sedation, seizures, and/or alcohol or other drug/substance intoxication.[3,7,8] Also, brain imaging studies may not be available, or may be initially interpreted as negative, in patients having a primary diagnosis of SCI. Symptoms, signs, and neuroimaging data important in the diagnosis of TBI in SCI patients are discussed in the next section.

DIAGNOSIS

Patients having an SCI should be assessed for the possibility of a co-occurring TBI on admission to a rehabilitation program. NIDRR SCI Model Systems started collecting data on associated TBI in 2011 due to the common occurrence of dual diagnosis.[11] A dual diagnosis of SCI with a severe TBI is usually established during acute care and is also usually obvious based on history and initial trauma neuroimaging studies. A dual diagnosis of SCI with a mild or moderate TBI may sometimes be overlooked during acute care especially in the case of co-occurring MTBI. MTBI, which is a synonym for concussion, accounts for as many as 80% of brain injuries that includes the spectrum of mild uncomplicated concussion to complicated concussion bordering on a moderately severe TBI.[8]

A diagnosis of MTBI and moderate TBI may be established during acute care prior to inpatient rehabilitation transfer in patients in which there was documentation of an

Table 1
Standard classifications of TBI severity

TBI Severity	Mild	Mild Complicated	Moderate	Severe
Initial Confusion or AMS	Documented or by history	Documented or by history	Documented or by history	Documented or by history
Initial GCS scores	13 to 15	13 to 15	9 to 12	3 to 8
PTA duration	<24 h	<24 h	<1 wk	>1 wk
LOC	If any, <1 h	If any, <1 h	Yes	Yes
Neuroimaging findings	No	Yes	Yes	Yes

Data from Refs.[3–5,7,8]

initial GCS score of 13 to 15 for MTBI or 9 to 12 for moderate TBI, pathology noted on the initial brain CT scan, known LOC, and/or PTA.[8,12] Due to the subtle nature of the initial symptoms and the often negative findings on emergency department brain CT scans and neurologic examination, however, especially in association with more pressing life-threatening traumatic injuries that include the SCI, diagnosis of an MTBI is often missed. Also, radiologic findings consistent with mild and moderate TBIs, in particular findings of contusions, may be missed in up to 67% of scans, especially when the scans are read by inexperienced radiologists.[13]

Brain injuries, especially concussions/MTBIs, may not become evident until an SCI patient is transferred to an inpatient rehabilitation unit. Individuals having a mild or moderate TBI may present on the inpatient rehabilitation unit with symptoms (listed in **Box 1**). A diagnosis of a mild or moderate TBI may be made on the inpatient rehabilitation unit in symptomatic patients based on review of the patient's history if there was evidence for confusion or LOC at the scene of trauma or subsequent PTA. Brain MRI studies may reveal findings consistent with TBI in patients with symptoms or clinical signs of brain injury but having otherwise negative brain CT scans.

EVALUATION

It is important for a dual diagnosis to be made in SCI patients having a co-occurring TBI so that the associated physical, cognitive, and behavioral symptoms are treated appropriately and so that the specialized rehabilitation is done accordingly. Cognitive and/or behavioral symptoms from a missed diagnosis of TBI during inpatient rehabilitation may be perceived by interdisciplinary staff, including physicians, nurses, therapists, and case managers, as noncompliance, inability to learn, maladaptive reactions to SCI, and poor motivation.[1,2,7] Also there are multiple potentially life-threatening and/or quality-of-life–threatening complications of TBI that also may be missed if a dual diagnosis is not made.

The evaluation should start with a thorough review of acute care records looking for any documentation of LOC, GCS scores, PTA duration, confusion, behavioral issues, seizures and/or abnormal results of any brain imaging studies. Special attention

---

Box 1
Possible symptoms of mild and moderate TBIs

- Headaches
- Dizziness
- Insomnia
- Imbalance/incoordination
- Emotional irritability/lability
- Depression/anxiety
- Impaired memory
- Executive dysfunction
- Behavioral manifestations
- Focal weakness/numbness
- Visual Impairments
- Impaired communication

should be given to review of paramedic/emergency rescue reports, acute care emergency department documentation, intensive care unit notes, consultation reports from all specialists, therapy notes, nursing notes, attending physician notes, and any psychology reports. The likelihood of a dual diagnosis may approach 60% when there is history of cervical spine trauma, a motor vehicle accident, or a fall from a significant height.[1–5] There usually is no clear documentation of durations of LOC or of PTA or GCS scores in most cases of an undocumented TBI diagnosis. PTA duration may be estimated by the interval of time to a patient's ability to consistently form new memories from day to day. Resolution of PTA usually occurs simultaneously with recovery from confusion/disorientation and is often preceded by the ability to consistently follow simple commands by a few weeks. Initial TBI severity may be determined by PTA durations (see **Table 1**).

Physical, behavioral, and cognitive symptoms and signs of brain injury in SCI patients may also be observed and reported by family members, interdisciplinary therapy staff and/or by the patient.

NEUROIMAGING

Patients who are having symptoms or signs of a mild or moderate TBI who may have had an initial negative brain CT scan may have abnormalities on brain MRI scans for up to 2 to 3 months after trauma, including findings consistent with areas of axonal shear injury and/or small contusions or hemorrhages.[14,15] Unilateral or multifocal lesions on MRI, particularly in the temporal or frontal lobes, are associated with neuropsychological symptoms in TBI.[8,14,15] Lesions of deep brain structures, such as the thalamus or multiple portions of the corpus callosum, are associated with moderate to severe brain injuries.[16] Isolated lesions of the posterior part of the corpus callosum can occur, however, in MTBI.[17]

Also, diffusion tensor MRI may be useful in showing specific brain motor pathway lesions that could be contributing to motor weakness resulting from TBI in patients with SCI.[18] Awareness of weakness related to TBI may assist clinicians in planning physical and occupational therapy rehabilitation strategies of dual diagnosis patients.

In addition, a brain CT scan is advisable in cases of SCI in which TBI is suspected if there had been no initial brain neuroimaging performed. Brain CT scan imaging is generally more effective than MRI in showing areas of skull fracture and other signs of acute trauma.

COMPLICATIONS
Head/Neck Trauma

Head and neck structures are often injured in association with cervical SCI and/or TBI. Associated head and neck structure injuries may be missed during acute care and initially present during rehabilitation with various symptoms and signs that may require special treatment; sometimes the symptoms of head/neck trauma are the presenting symptoms of the co-occurring TBI.

Fractures at the skull base or frontal bone
Fractures at the skull base or frontal bone may be associated with dural membrane lacerations, which may present as a cerebrospinal fluid (CSF) fistula leak and patient complaint of a chronic running nose or fluid in an ear. Trauma to the frontal bone frequently involves the paranasal sinuses and may result in CSF leakage from the nose (rhinorrhea) and pneumocephalus that may cause headaches; these fractures may also involve the orbit. Fractures involving the middle and posterior skull base

often involve the petrous portion of the temporal bone and are associated with risk for facial palsy, hearing loss, and CSF fistulas that leak from the ears (otorrhea). Work-up should include skull radiographs or brain CT scan. Neurosurgical consultation is required if CSF fistula is suspected because there is significant associated risk for the development of an intracranial infection.

Orbital fractures

Orbital fractures may result in diplopia secondary to opthalmoplegia associated with traumatic neuropathies of cranial nerves 3, 4, and/or 6; or due to entrapments of the muscles of eye movement. Diplopia may also occur from vascular trauma or injury of central pathways directly related to brain injury.

Temporal bone fractures

Temporal bone fractures may be associated with traumatic neuropathies of cranial nerves 7 and/or 8 and may present with ipsilateral facial palsy, hearing loss, and/or vertigo. Vertigo/dizziness is also the second most common postconcussion symptom after headache and often occurs in the absence of skull fractures (discussed later).[8]

Vascular trauma

Vascular trauma, such as dissections and fistulas involving the anterior and posterior blood supply to the head and neck, including the extracranial and intracranial branches of the vertebral and carotid arteries, may present with symptoms and signs that include neck pain, unilateral headache or facial pain, and transient or fixed neurologic findings referable to specific brain vascular territories. Trauma is a primary cause of carotid cavernous fistulas and the cavernous sinus syndrome, which may present with diplopia, unilateral facial pain, and/or numbness, Horner syndrome, and unilateral scleral erythema.

Eye injuries

Eye injuries may occur, especially in association with frontal impact head trauma and orbital fractures. Vision impairment may directly result from trauma of eye structures and/or extraocular muscles or from indirect injury, such as exposure keratopathy, due to incomplete lid closure and inadequate eye lubrication after a traumatic facial palsy.

Postconcussion Syndrome

The postconcussion syndrome is a complex of somatic, affective, and cognitive symptoms that is well described in the medical literature, which may complicate the recovery after a TBI, which may be a presenting feature of TBI, and which may result from brain injury or from trauma involving other head/neck structures.[8] The most common symptoms are headache and dizziness followed by impaired sleep, neck pain, hearing loss, and emotional and/or cognitive problems. The neuropsychological problems may pose an important challenge in the rehabilitation of dual diagnosis patients.

Headache

Headache is usually peripheral in origin rather than due to central nervous system causes and may also result from the effect of various medications. In dual diagnosis patients with cervical spine injury, radiculopathy involving the second and/ or third nerve root may cause headaches.[19] In patients with posttraumatic dizziness, headache may be due to inner ear injuries, such as benign positional vertigo or a perilymphatic fistula.[8] Possible central causes of posttraumatic headache include pneumocephalus, CSF fistulas, and chronic extra-axial fluid collections, such as a subdural hematoma or hygroma. Neuroimaging studies and/or neurologic consultation should be considered when headaches interfere with rehabilitation progress.

Dizziness
Dizziness is usually peripheral in origin rather than due to central nervous system causes and may also result from the effect of various medications. The most common posttraumatic cause is benign positional vertigo due to inner ear injury.[8] In dual diagnosis patients with cervical spine injury, dizziness may be related to the cervical spine trauma.[20]

Hearing loss
Hearing loss may be due to neural or conductive injury. Conductive causes include tympanic membrane rupture, ossicle disruption, or a middle ear hematoma. Hearing loss related to neural injury of cranial nerve 8 often occurs in association with temporal bone skull fractures and/or vestibular injury.

Sleep impairment
Sleep impairment is common in TBI and SCI patients and may be multifactorial in etiology. Chronic pain, anxiety, and/or depression may be causes. Impaired sleep may interfere with rehabilitation progress.

Neck pain
Neck pain is especially common when the mechanism of trauma involved a motor vehicle accident in which there was hyperflexion and hyperextension of the neck. In addition to cervical SCI, other associated pathologic findings may include torn muscles or ligaments, vertebral column fractures, radiculopathy, and occasionally a Horner syndrome from cervical sympathetic pathway involvement.

Neuropsychological symptoms
Neuropsychological symptoms, including emotional and/or cognitive impairments, in a dual diagnosis patient may sometimes be the presenting feature of a TBI. Emotional symptoms may include irritability, lability, anxiety, and depression. Cognitive symptoms may include difficulties with concentration, attention, memory, word finding/speech, perception, information processing, and executive functions.

Neuropsychological symptoms in dual diagnosis patients may result from brain injury and/or may be related to nonorganic factors. Patients with unilateral or multifocal brain lesions on neuroimaging studies are more likely to have neuropsychological symptoms as a result of brain trauma.[8,14,15] Emotional symptoms unrelated to brain injury may stem from the subjective experience of somatic problems, such as pain, cognitive difficulties, or adjustment issues related to the trauma.[8] Cognitive symptoms unrelated to brain injury may occur from distracted concentration/attention due to anxiety, depression, or somatic problems, including pain.[8]

Seizures

The risk of posttraumatic epilepsy increases with worsening brain injury severity, intracerebral hematoma, cortical contusions, depressed skull fractures, and/or seizures that occur after the first week after trauma, in which case anticonvulsant medication prophylaxis is warranted. A preexisting poorly controlled seizure disorder or a previously undiagnosed seizure disorder may sometimes be the source of a seizure that contributed to the trauma that resulted in dual diagnosis TBI/SCI.

Complications in Dual Diagnosis with Moderate–Severe TBI

Complications in moderate–severe TBI in dual diagnosis patients may be life threatening or quality-of-life threatening and may manifest during the acute care hospitalization or instead may sometimes be initially diagnosed during rehabilitation. Potential complications of moderate–severe TBI may include physical, cognitive/behavioral, metabolic, and posttraumatic complications (**Box 2**). Rehabilitation challenges posed by some of these physical, cognitive, and emotional problems are also discussed in the following section.

Common physical factors that may inhibit motor recovery in TBI/SCI may include heterotopic ossification (HO) and/or spasticity. HO may occur in 10% to 70% of patients with a solitary diagnosis of TBI or SCI, but the risk increases in patients with a dual diagnosis, spasticity, prolonged immobility prior to rehabilitation, a long bone fracture, and/or history of posttraumatic coma greater than 2 weeks.[21] Common locations are soft tissues areas around the hips, elbows, and knees; symptoms include pain, heat, swelling, and loss of range-of-motion in the areas affected. SCI patients may not report discomfort or pain. Bisphosphonates and surgical excision may be the most effective treatments.[21] Prevention includes early passive range-of-motion exercises, nonsteroidal anti-inflammatory medications, and treatment of spasticity.[21]

Spasticity occurs as a result of posttraumatic lesions affecting upper motor neuron pathways in the brain and/or spinal cord and is common in dual diagnosis patients with moderate to severe brain injuries and/or cervical or thoracic spine trauma. Manifestations of spasticity may include muscle stiffness, spasms, pain/discomfort, and

---

Box 2
Possible complications in moderate–severe TBI with SCI

- Neuroendocrine dysfunction
- Disorders of sodium regulation
  - Excess ADH/hyponatremia
  - Low ADH/hypernatremia–DI
- Obstructive hydrocephalus
- Paroxysmal sympathetic hyperactivity/sympathetic storming
- Spasticity
- HO
- Impaired arousal/apathy
- Agitation/aggression
- Impaired cognition/perception
- Seizures/epilepsy
- Oropharyngeal dysphagia
- Aspiration pneumonia
- Bulbar impairments
- Sensorimotor impairments
- Communication impairments
- Apraxia/cognitive-motor disorder
- Depression/anxiety

associated functional impairments affecting mobility and the performance of activities of daily living. Spasticity also increases the risk for the development of HO,[21] contractures, and skin ulcerations. The management of spasticity in dual diagnosis patients represents a challenge because some of the medications may have side effects affecting the recovery of cognition and memory in TBI and/or may lead to loss of function, particularly when spasticity is counterbalancing the effects of paresis in SCI. Treatment options of spasticity may include physical, pharmacologic, and surgical options (summarized in **Table 2**).[22–26]

Table 2
Summary of spasticity management options

Treatment Options	Actions	Side Effects
Physical interventions stretching, splinting, bracing, casting, etc	Improvement of range of motion, flexibility	Inadvertent injury to muscle or connective tissue, or fractures
Electrical stimulation	Dermatome/afferent feedback; stimulation of antagonist muscles	May include discomfort, possible cardiac arrhythmia?
Baclofen	Binds to the γ-aminobutyric acid (GABA) receptors in spinal cord; decreases stretch reflexes	May include muscle weakness, sedation, dizziness, withdrawal syndrome
Tizanidine	Central α_2-adrenergic receptor agonist	May include sedation, weakness, dizziness, elevation of liver enzymes
Diazepam	Facilitates the postsynaptic action of GABA	May include sedation, cognitive impairment, dizziness, potential for dependence, withdrawal syndrome
Dantrolene	Reduces the release of calcium into the sarcoplasmic reticulum of muscles	May include muscle weakness, sedation, hepatotoxicity
Clonidine	Central-acting α_2-adrenergic agonist	May include hypotension, bradycardia, dizziness, constipation
Gabapentin	Exact actions unknown, blocks voltage-dependent calcium channels modulating excitatory neurotransmitter release	May include sedation, dizziness
Intrathecal baclofen pump	See Baclofen entry.	May include risk for infection, overdose, or withdrawal
Botulinum toxin injection	Acts at the neuromuscular junction blocking acetylcholine release	May include weakness in target muscles and/or other proximal muscles
Surgical procedures (such as dorsal rhizotomy, myelotomy, cordotomy)	Surgical lesion of neural pathway contributing to hypertonicity	May include various neurosurgical complications; weakness, sensory loss, scoliosis

Data from Refs.[22–26]

Dysphagia, due to mechanical, obstructive, or neurologic problems, is another complication that frequently occurs in moderate to severe TBIs as well as SCIs. The likelihood of dysphagia increases in SCI patients having upper cervical spine trauma, older age, tracheostomy, ventilation, and cervical surgery that may include anterior and/or posterior instrumentation or occipital-cervical fusion procedures.[27,28] Dysphagia is likely in TBI patients having tracheostomy, history of ventilation greater than 2 weeks, Rancho Los Amigos (RLAS) level 6 or less, previous neuroimaging showing midline shift or brainstem lesions, and/or intracranial pathology that required emergency surgery.[29,30] Dual diagnosis patients having history of intubation may sometimes have secondary mechanical injury to vocal cords causing dysphagia. Obstructive impairments of swallowing may occur as a complication of cervical spine surgeries that cause an abnormal cervical lordosis and/or oropharyngeal stenosis. Central nervous system causes of dysphagia may include lesions affecting cortical, subcortical, and brainstem sensory or motor pathways involved in swallowing.[31] Dual diagnosis patients having any of the risk factors previously cited should be evaluated for dysphagia on admission to an inpatient rehabilitation unit. A modified barium swallow study is the diagnostic procedure that may be performed to confirm a swallowing disorder.[32] There are multiple treatment options for mechanical, obstructive, and neurologic causes of dysphagia; however, impairments of cognition and/or behavior (discussed later) pose a special challenge to the therapeutic approach.

Dual diagnosis patients with moderate to severe TBI are at a high risk for having psychopathology that my include adjustment disorders and neuropsychiatric and cognitive problems, such as depression, anxiety, agitation, aggression, impulsive behavior, impaired memory, impaired attention/concentration, and sleep disturbances.[7,33–37] Neuropsychiatric and cognitive problems are likely in patients having lesions involving the frontal and/or temporal lobes, amygdala, and limbic system.[8,33,35] Agitation, aggression and restlessness are especially likely in TBI patients that are at level 4 on the RLAS cognitive scale.[38] Although the pharmacologic management of agitation, aggression and restlessness in TBI remains controversial, there is some consensus of opinion that β-blocker medications may be useful.[37] Similarly, the pharmacologic management of impaired concentration, attention, and speed of information processing remains controversial but there is some consensus of opinion that methylphenidate may be useful.[37] Pharmacologic management options for neurobehavioral and cognitive disorders after TBI are summarized in **Table 3**.[33–37] Nonpharmacologic therapeutic strategies for the management of psychopathology in dual diagnosis patients are discussed later.

Metabolic problems, including disorders of serum sodium regulation and/or neuroendocrine dysfunction, may occur in dual diagnosis patients having moderate–severe TBI, particularly when a lesion involves the hypothalamic-pituitary brain pathways.[39–46] Hyponatremia may occur from the syndrome of inappropriate antidiuretic hormone secretion (SIADH) or from cerebral salt-wasting syndrome (CSWS).[40–43] In SIADH, there is normovolemic to hypervolemic hyponatremia due to the dilution of serum sodium concentration from renal water retention and sodium excretion caused by excessive release of antidiuretic hormone (ADH) by the hypothalamus.[40–43] In CSWS, there is hypovolemic hyponatremia from excessive renal excretion of both water and sodium resulting in dehydration that is caused by disruption of hypothalamic-pituitary pathways that stimulate adrenal release of cortisol.[40–43] SIADH is treated with sodium supplementation, fluid restriction, and sometimes mineralocorticoids. CSWS is treated with sodium supplementation, hydration, and mineralocorticoids.[40–43] Untreated, profound hyponatremia can result in encephalopathy and seizures. Although less common, diabetes insipidus (DI) may also occur when TBI results in inadequate or

Table 3
Medication options for mood disorders and agitation/aggression

Medication	Purpose	Possible Side Effects
Benzodiazepines (lorazepam, diazepam clonazepam...)	Acute management of agitation	May include sedation, impaired cognition, muscle weakness...
Anticonvulsants (valproate, carbamazepine, lamotrigine...)	Agitation/(Seizure prophylaxis)	May include sedation, thrombocytopenia, hepatotoxicity...
Antipsychotics (haloperidol, quetiapine, ziprasidone...)	Temporary agitation management	May include slow motor recovery, prolonged PTA, extrapyramidal syndrome...
Amantadine	May enhance cognition, concentration, attention and decrease agitation	May include decreased seizure threshold
Methylphenidate	May enhance cognition, concentration, attention, memory and decrease agitation	May include tachycardia, hypertension, headache, rash...
β-blockers (propranolol, pindolol)	Agitation treatment	May include orthostatic hypotension...
Tricyclic antidepressants (amitriptyline, desipramine, doxepin, imipramine)	Depression, agitation, sleep	May include decreased seizure threshold
Sertraline	Depression, agitation	May include suicidal ideation, withdrawal symptoms, birth defects...
Buspirone	Depression, agitation	May include dizziness, headache, insomnia...
Lithium	Severe agitation/aggression, may reduce need for antipsychotics	May include thirst, weight gain, tremor, seizures, renal and neural toxicity...

Data from Refs.[33–37]

absent secretion of ADH, which causes excessive renal loss of free water causing dehydration with hypernatremia.[43] DI may present clinically with polydipsia, polyuria, and encephalopathy. It may be treated with ADH, which is also known as vasopressin. Other central neuroendocrine problems that may inhibit recovery in dual diagnosis patients include hypothyroidism, adrenal insufficiency, hypogonadism, and impaired secretion of growth hormone.[1,44–46]

The most common posttraumatic complications in dual diagnosis patients with moderate–severe TBI are seizures and obstructive hydrocephalus. Seizures are discussed previously. Risk factors for development of obstructive hydrocephalus requiring permanent placement of a ventricular-peritoneal (VP) shunt include severe TBI, older age, prior ventriculostomy, craniotomy within 48 hours of trauma, and prior culture-positive CSF.[47–50] Patients who reach a plateau in functional progress or demonstrate clinical regression or signs of worsening encephalopathy and cognitive impairments should be evaluated with neuroimaging studies for obstructive hydrocephalus and/or a prior VP shunt malfunction.

REHABILITATION

TBI may limit the rate and degree of functional progress during various phases of rehabilitation in SCI patients; however, this limitation effect is not linear with TBI severity but is instead affected by multiple factors.[6] In general, the best functional recovery may be expected in paraplegic patients with co-occurring mild or moderate TBI where acute rehabilitation motor/cognitive outcomes may be equivalent in comparison to those of paraplegic patients without TBI.[5] Delayed and/or suboptimal motor skill acquisition is more likely in paraplegic patients with severe TBI due to impaired cognition.[5] Laterality of brain hemisphere lesions in moderate TBI may affect motor recovery in incomplete cervical SCI patients.[1]

Rehabilitation strategies for the management of dual diagnosis patients with moderate–severe TBI during the confused/agitated to automatic/appropriate stages of cognitive recovery are provided in **Boxes 3** and **4**. In general, young previously healthy patients with a moderate–severe TBI should gradually improve in both cognitive and

---

Box 3
Rehabilitation strategies in moderate–severe TBI with SCI for the confused/agitated patient

- Provide private room near nurse station
- Restraints only when necessary for safety
- Covering brace and feeding tube with shirt/abdominal binder lessen agitation and risk for inadvertent removal
- If possible, full-time attendant care
- Minimize schedule disruptions/overstimulation/distractions
  - Regular nursing care, including catheterizations
  - Regular therapy schedule at times of day when most alert
- Maintain appropriate sleep-wake cycles
  - Avoid daytime sedation
  - Use medication at night to limit restlessness/agitation
- Tilt-in-space wheelchair for pressure relief minimizes agitation
- Frequent reorientation by staff
- Therapy recommendations
  - Cotreatment with 1 therapist giving instructions each session
  - Patient instructions should be short 1-step commands
  - Rest breaks to avoid fatigue/frustration; fatigue ends session
  - Therapy to occur at times of day when patient is most alert
  - Therapy to be provided in a nondistracting quiet area
  - Aggressive/inappropriate behavior to be dealt with firmly/instantly
  - Successes to be rewarded with positive feedback
  - Involve psychology for patient/family support/therapy
- Educate family on TBI/SCI, short/long-term goals and their role

Data from Somner JL, Witkiewicz PM. The therapeutic challenges of dual diagnosis: TBI/SCI. Brain Inj 2004;18(12):1297–308.

Box 4
Rehabilitation strategies in moderate–severe TBI with SCI for the confused/nonagitated patient

Confused/nonagitated/inappropriate

- Therapy sessions still best in quiet area of gym
- Patients respond well to structure and redirection for task completion
- Now able to consistently follow 1- and 2-step commands
- Patients still benefit from rest breaks and avoidance of overstimulation
- Full-time supervision by staff or caregivers still important

Confused/appropriate to automatic/appropriate

- Therapy may now focus more on SCI rehabilitation interventions
- Therapy may occur in open gym
- Orientation group, memory logbook, and signs in room helpful
- Checklists and environmental cues useful in planning/initiating necessary SCI activities, such as pressure relief and catheterizations
- Patient should eventually learn and verbalize why braces and treatments are necessary
- Paraparetic should learn to don/doff braces, dress in bed, wheelchair mobility
- Family education (including all care, such as bladder care)
- Including patient and family in support group is helpful

Data from Somner JL, Witkiewicz PM. The therapeutic challenges of dual diagnosis: TBI/SCI. Brain Inj 2004;18(12):1297–308.

---

emotional function, allowing for better tolerance and efficacy of SCI rehabilitation interventions.

Dual diagnosis patients with moderate–severe TBI who reach a plateau in functional progress or who regress may have a posttraumatic, metabolic, physical, cognitive, or emotional complication (see **Box 2**). Functional regression or clinical deterioration may occur with TBI-related neuroendocrine dysfunction, disorders of sodium regulation, depression, or the development of obstructive hydrocephalus or a vetriculoperitoneal shunt malfunction.

SUMMARY

Any patient having an SCI should be assessed for the possibility of a co-occurring TBI on admission to a rehabilitation program because a dual diagnosis is common and it complicates management and expected outcomes. Incidence of concomitant TBI with SCI may approach 60% when risk factors include motor vehicle collision, fall, and/or alcohol intoxication as the cause of trauma, complete SCI level, and a C1–C4 level of injury.[1–5]

Diagnosis of mild–moderate severity TBIs may be missed during acute care hospitalizations of SCI, especially when there was need for sedation or intubation and/or the presence of acute trauma-related life-threatening issues. Cognitive and/or behavioral symptoms from a missed diagnosis may be perceived during rehabilitation as noncompliance, inability to learn, maladaptive reactions to SCI, and poor motivation[1,2,7]; and, there are life-threatening and/or quality-of-life threatening complications of TBI that also may be missed if a dual diagnosis is not made.

Expected rate and degree of functional progress during various phases of rehabilitation in SCI patients are often limited by a co-occurring TBI. A plateau in functional recovery or clinical regression may be due to a posttraumatic, metabolic, physical, cognitive, or emotional complication.

REFERENCES

1. Inoue T, Lin A, Ma X, et al. Combined SCI and TBI: recovery of forelimb function after unilateral cervical spinal cord injury (SCI) is retarded by contralateral traumatic brain injury (TBI), and ipsilateral TBI balances the effects of SCI on paw placement. Exp Neurol 2013;248:136–47.
2. Somner JL, Witkiewicz PM. The therapeutic challenges of dual diagnosis: TBI/SCI. Brain Inj 2004;18(12):1297–308.
3. Macciocci S, Seel RT, Thompson N, et al. Spinal cord injury and co-occuring traumatic brain injury: assessment and incidence. Arch Phys Med Rehabil 2008;89(7):1350–7.
4. Hagen EM, Eide GE, Rekand T, et al. Traumatic spinal cord injury and concomitant brain injury: a cohort study. Acta Neurol Scand Suppl 2010; 190:51–7.
5. Macciocchi S, Seel RT, Warshowsky A, et al. Co-occurring traumatic brain injury and acute spinal cord injury rehabilitation outcomes. Arch Phys Med Rehabil 2012;93(10):1788–94.
6. Macciocchi SN, Bowman B, Coker J, et al. Effect of co-morbid traumatic brain injury on functional outcome of persons with spinal cord injuries. Am J Phys Med Rehabil 2004;83(1):22–6.
7. Bradbury CL, Wodchis WP, Mikulis DJ, et al. Traumatic brain injury in patients with traumatic spinal cord injury: clinical and economic consequences. Arch Phys Med Rehabil 2008;89(12 Suppl):S77–84.
8. Kushner D. Mild traumatic brain injury: toward understanding manifestations and treatment. Arch Intern Med 1998;158:1617–24.
9. American Spinal Injury Association (ASIA). Standards for neurological and functional classification of spinal cord injury. Chicago: The Association; 1992.
10. National Data and Statistical Center. Traumatic brain injury model systems. Online syllabus. Available at: http://www.tbindsc.org/syllabus.aspx. Accessed September 5, 2013.
11. National Institute on Disabilities Rehabilitation and Research, Spinal Cord Injury Model Systems. SCI model systems form 2011-2016. Available at: https://www.nscisc.uab.edu/PublicDocuments/dat. Accessed September 5, 2013.
12. Ryu WH, Feinstein A, Colantonio A, et al. Early identification and incidence of mild TBI in Ontario. Can J Neurol Sci 2009;36(4):429–35.
13. Laalo JP, Kurki TJ, Sonninen PH, et al. Reliability of diagnosis of traumatic brain injury by computed tomography in the acute phase. J Neurotrauma 2009; 26(12):2169–78.
14. Levin HS, Williams DH, Eisenberg HM, et al. Serial MRI and neurobehavioral findings after mild to moderate closed head injury. J Neurol Neurosurg Psychiatry 1992;55:255–62.
15. Levin HS, Amparo E, Eisenberg HM, et al. Magnetic resonance imaging and computerized tomography in relation to the neurobehavioral sequelae after mild and moderate closed head injuries. J Neurosurg 1987;66:706–13.
16. Bigler ED, Maxwell WL. Neuroimaging and neuropathology of TBI. NeuroRehabilitation 2011;28(2):63–74. http://dx.doi.org/10.3233/NRE-2011-0633.

17. Aoki Y, Inokuchi R, Gunshin M, et al. Diffusion tensor imaging studies of mild traumatic brain injury: a meta-analysis. J Neurol Neurosurg Psychiatry 2012; 83(9):870–6.

18. Choi GS, Kim OL, Kim SH, et al. Classification of cause of motor weakness in traumatic brain injury using diffusion tensor imaging. Arch Neurol 2012;69(3): 363–7.

19. Wilson PR. Chronic neck pain and cervicogenic headache. Clin J Pain 1991;7: 5–11.

20. Hinoki M. Vertigo due to whiplash injury: a neurological approach. Acta Otolaryngol Suppl 1985;419:9–29.

21. Aubut JA, Mehta S, Cullen N, et al. A comparison of heterotopic ossification treatment within the traumatic brain and spinal cord injured population: an evidence based systematic review. NeuroRehabilitation 2011;28(2):151–60.

22. Hsieh JT, Connolly S, Townson AF, et al. Spasticity after spinal cord injury: an evidence-based review of current interventions. Top Spinal Cord Inj Rehabil 2007;13(1):81–97.

23. Adams MM, Hicks AL. Spasticity after spinal cord injury. Spinal Cord 2005; 43(10):577–86.

24. Zafonte R, Elovic EP, Lombard L. Acute care management of post-TBI spasticity. J Head Trauma Rehabil 2004;19(2):89–100.

25. Thompson AJ, Jarrett L, Lockley L, et al. Clinical management of spasticity. J Neurol Neurosurg Psychiatry 2005;76:459–63.

26. Roberts A. Surgical management of spasticity. J Child Orthop 2013;7(5): 389–94.

27. Tian W, Yu J. The role of C2-C7 and O-C2 angle in the development of dysphagia after cervical spine surgery. Dysphagia 2013;28(2):131–8.

28. Kirshblum S, Johnston MV, Brown J, et al. Predictors of dysphagia after spinal cord injury. Arch Phys Med Rehabil 1999;80(9):1101–5.

29. Mackay LE, Morgan AS, Bernstein BA. Factors affecting oral feeding with severe traumatic brain injury. J Head Trauma Rehabil 1999;14(5):435–47.

30. Mackay LE, Morgan AS, Bernstein BA. Swallowing disorders in severe brain injury: risk factors affecting return to oral intake. Arch Phys Med Rehabil 1999; 80(4):365–71.

31. Kushner DS, Peters K, Eroglu ST, et al. Neuromuscular electrical stimulation efficacy in acute stroke feeding tube-dependent dysphagia during inpatient rehabilitation. Am J Phys Med Rehabil 2013;92(6):486–95.

32. Ott DJ, Pikna LA. Clinical and videofluoroscopic evaluation of swallowing disorders. AJR Am J Roentgenol 1993;161(3):507–13.

33. Jorge R, Robinson RG. Mood disorders following traumatic brain injury. Int Rev Psychiatry 2003;15(4):317–27.

34. Bhalerao SU, Geurtjens C, Thomas GR, et al. Understanding the neuropsychiatric consequences associated with significant traumatic brain injury. Brain Inj 2013;27(7–8):767–74.

35. Saoût V, Gambart G, Leguay D, et al. Aggressive behavior after traumatic brain injury. Ann Phys Rehabil Med 2011;54(4):259–69.

36. Chew E, Zafonte RD. Pharmacological management of neurobehavioral disorders following traumatic brain injury–a state-of-the-art review. J Rehabil Res Dev 2009;46(6):851–79.

37. Neurobehavioral Guidelines Working Group, Warden DL, Gordon B, et al. Guidelines for the pharmacologic treatment of neurobehavioral sequelae of traumatic brain injury. J Neurotrauma 2006;23(10):1468–501.

38. APPENDIX B: Rancho Los Amigos scale-revised. Continuum (Minneap Minn) 2011;17(3 Neurorehabilitation):646–8.

39. Schneider HJ, Kreitschmann-Andermahr I, Ghigo E, et al. Hypothalamopituitary dysfunction following traumatic brain injury and aneurysmal subarachnoid hemorrhage: a systematic review. JAMA 2007;298(12):1429–38.

40. Lohani S, Devkota UP. Hyponatremia in patients with traumatic brain injury: etiology, incidence, and severity correlation. World Neurosurg 2011;76(3–4): 355–60.

41. Harrigan MR. Cerebral salt wasting syndrome: a review. Neurosurgery 1996; 38(1):152–60.

42. Moro N, Katayama Y, Igarashi T, et al. Hyponatremia in patients with traumatic brain injury: incidence, mechanism, and response to sodium supplementation or retention therapy with hydrocortisone. Surg Neurol 2007;68(4):387–93.

43. Agha A, Sherlock M, Phillips J, et al. The natural history of post-traumatic neurohypophysial dysfunction. Eur J Endocrinol 2005;152(3):371–7.

44. Urban RJ, Harris P, Masel B. Anterior hypopituitarism following traumatic brain injury. Brain Inj 2005;19(5):349–58.

45. Aimaretti G, Ghigo E. Traumatic brain injury and hypopituitarism. ScientificWorldJournal 2005;5:777–81.

46. Ghigo E, Masel B, Aimaretti G, et al. Consensus guidelines on screening for hypopituitarism following traumatic brain injury. Brain Inj 2005;19(9):711–24.

47. Bauer DF, McGwin G Jr, Melton SM, et al. Risk factors for conversion to permanent ventricular shunt in patients receiving therapeutic ventriculostomy for traumatic brain injury. Neurosurgery 2011;68(1):85–8.

48. Kammersgaard LP, Linnemann M, Tibæk M. Hydrocephalus following severe traumatic brain injury in adults. Incidence, timing, and clinical predictors during rehabilitation. NeuroRehabilitation 2013;33(3):473–80.

49. Denes Z, Barsi P, Szel I, et al. Complication during postacute rehabilitation: patients with posttraumatic hydrocephalus. Int J Rehabil Res 2011;34(3):222–6.

50. Guyot LL, Michael DB. Post-traumatic hydrocephalus. Neurol Res 2000;22(1): 25–8.

Index

Note: Page numbers of article titles are in **boldface** type.

A

Acupuncture
in chronic neuropathic pain management after SCI, 559–560
Anticonvulsants
in chronic neuropathic pain management after SCI, 555
Antidepressants
in chronic neuropathic pain management after SCI, 555–556
Antispasticity agents
in chronic neuropathic pain management after SCI, 558

B

Baclofen
intrathecal
for SCI–related spasticity, **655–669**. *See also* Intrathecal baclofen (ITB), for SCI–related spasticity
Bacteriuria
UTIs in neurogenic bladder dysfunction related to, 606
Behavioral modification
in cardiometabolic disease in SCI management, 584–588
Bladder control
after SCI
FES in restoration of, 646–647
Breathing
physiology of, 620, 624–625

C

Cannabinoids
in chronic neuropathic pain management after SCI, 557
Cardiometabolic disease
in SCI
reducing of, **573–604**
behavioral modification in, 584–588
pharmacologic approaches to, 585, 589–596
therapeutic lifestyle interventions in, 574–585
diet-related, 576–580
exercise-related, 580–583
shoulder pain management, 584
risks associated with, 573–574
Catheterization
in UTI prevention in neurogenic bladder dysfunction
external catheters, 611

Phys Med Rehabil Clin N Am 25 (2014) 697–705
http://dx.doi.org/10.1016/S1047-9651(14)00073-4
1047-9651/14/$ – see front matter © 2014 Elsevier Inc. All rights reserved.

pmr.theclinics.com

Moving?

Make sure your subscription moves with you!

To notify us of your new address, find your **Clinics Account Number** (located on your mailing label above your name), and contact customer service at:

Email: journalscustomerservice-usa@elsevier.com

800-654-2452 (subscribers in the U.S. & Canada)
314-447-8871 (subscribers outside of the U.S. & Canada)

Fax number: 314-447-8029

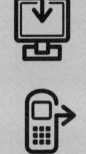

Elsevier Health Sciences Division
Subscription Customer Service
3251 Riverport Lane
Maryland Heights, MO 63043

*To ensure uninterrupted delivery of your subscription, please notify us at least 4 weeks in advance of move.

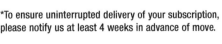
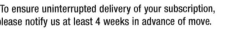

Printed and bound by CPI Group (UK) Ltd, Croydon, CR0 4YY

03/10/2024

01040488-0002